CW00742441

How to Heal Family Trauma

Simple Techniques to Free Yourself from Inherited Wounds, Let Go of the Emotional Baggage of the Past, and Create a Positive Future, without Guilt

Logan Mind

A Gift for You!

Emotional Intelligence for Social Success

Here's what you'll find in the **book**:

• Proven techniques to enhance your **emotional intelligence**

• Strategies for effective **communication** and building strong **relationships**

• Tips for managing **emotions** in various social situations

Just click or follow the link below to start experiencing greater social **success**:

https://pxl.to/loganmindfreebook

Download your 3 FREE EXTRAS too!

These extras are a great complementary **resource** to help you delve deeper into the concepts covered in your free book and to support your journey towards enhanced emotional intelligence and social success.

The extras are:

• A downloadable and practical PDF 21-Day **Challenge** for the book

• 101+ Messages of Self-Love and Compassion

• Identifying and Breaking Negative Patterns

Just click or follow the link below to gain instant access to the extras:

https://pxl.to/9-hthfft-lm-extras

Help Me!

When you're done reading, I need your help to make a difference.

When you support an independent author, you're supporting a dream.

If you enjoyed reading this book, please take a moment to leave an **honest review** by visiting the link below. Your feedback not only guides future readers but also helps me grow as a writer.

• **Your reviews matter!**

• They provide valuable insights.

• They help reach a broader audience.

If you have suggestions for improvements, you can contact me via the email you'll find at the link below. Alternatively, you can scan the QR code to get directly to the feedback page.

It only takes **a few seconds**, but your voice has a **huge impact** on my journey.

Visit this link to leave feedback:

https://pxl.to/9-hthfft-lm-review

Join my Review Team!

Thank you for reading my **book**! I'd love to invite you to join my **Review Team**. If you're an **avid reader**, you can receive a free copy of my book in exchange for your **honest feedback**. This would be extremely helpful for me.

Here's how you can join the ARC team:

• Click on "Join Review Team"

• Sign Up to BookSprout

• Get notified every time I release a new **book**

Check out the team at this link:

https://pxl.to/loganmindteam

Introduction

Ever **wondered** why some family dynamics just seem off? Like there's an invisible script everyone's following, filled with **conflicts** you can't quite put your finger on? Well, that's exactly what this book aims to solve.

Think about it. Family drama isn't just your parents being overbearing or siblings being annoying. It goes much deeper than that. This book uncovers how wounds aren't only physical; they can be **emotional** scars handed down through generations. Like a sad family heirloom. And guess what? You're not alone in carrying this burden. Anxieties. Fears. Relational hiccups. They can all tie back to past family **traumas** that you didn't even cause.

So why am I the one here telling you about it? Over the years, I've learned a lot about human behavior and the ways different people connect (or fail to). My journey isn't just limited to writing; I've worked closely with folks from varied backgrounds — from business execs to everyday people struggling with their own stories. Whether through coaching sessions or group activities, I've seen firsthand the profound **impact** that unresolved family stuff can have on our lives.

Ever heard about things like epigenetics and trauma transmission? It's science telling us that trauma can affect not just you but also the next generations. Fascinating, right? Addressing this familial weight isn't just a tick-box exercise. It's a deep-rooted necessity vital for carving out a better future for yourself.

You might find yourself thinking, "But my family didn't go through any major drama, so why do I need this?" Here's the kicker. Trauma isn't just about big, shocking events. It can be subtle. Silent judgments. Comparisons. Expectations. You don't even realize when these patterns creep into your psyche, shaping your decisions, **relationships**, and even your happiness. Yeah, it's a complex beast.

And concern over straining family ties can hold you back from addressing these issues. You're scared it might make holidays awkward or create rifts that weren't there before. Been there. But restrained silence isn't the solution. This book teaches sensitive ways to approach these tough subjects and even provides terminologies to give shape to these feelings.

Okay, that's your daily dose of heavy thoughts. But let's look at the positive side. Imagine breaking free from those ugly cycles of guilt and inherited stress. Picture crafting relationships full of meaningful connections. To know that the person you see in the mirror isn't haunted by a past you can't control but is guided by a hopeful and empowering narrative. That's the gift this book promises.

In conclusion, getting into these pages isn't just about understanding family or overcoming the debris left by trauma. It's about rewriting your own story. A story that doesn't cling to inherited emotional baggage but celebrates abundant possibilities. So buckle up, my friend. You're on the verge of discovering how freeing it is to forge a new **narrative** — without guilt.

Ready for it? This book is your map to a world of **healing** and happiness that you deserve.

Chapter 1: Understanding Family Trauma

Ever wonder why some things seem to run in the family but aren't physical features? That's what I asked myself before starting this book. Do you ever feel like you're carrying **weight** that's not yours? In this chapter, we'll unpack the hidden **burdens** passed down through generations.

You might be surprised to spot signs of **inherited** trauma you didn't even realize you had. Does it mess with your **well-being** or relationships? Absolutely. But here's the kicker—to fix the cycle, you've got to know it exists. By the end, you'll be more **aware** and prepared to make a change.

Family **trauma** can be sneaky, affecting you in ways you might not expect. It can shape your **behavior**, influence your choices, and even impact how you interact with others. The good news? Once you recognize these patterns, you're already on the path to breaking free from them.

Think about it—have you ever noticed yourself repeating **habits** or reactions that feel oddly familiar, almost as if they've been programmed into you? That's not by chance. These could be echoes of experiences your family has gone through, silently passed down to you.

Ready to dive deeper? This chapter will help you connect the dots between your family's past and your present. You'll gain insights into how generational experiences shape who you are and how you navigate the world.

Keen to find out how to start your **transformation**? Buckle up—this is where the journey begins. By understanding family trauma, you're taking the first step towards healing not just yourself, but potentially breaking the cycle for future generations. Let's get started!

The Nature of Family Trauma

Alright, let's dive into this. Family **trauma** is when bad experiences ripple through the whole family. It's more than just one person feeling down—it's like everyone in the family gets caught in this web of pain. When you go through something really tough, like abuse or neglect, it doesn't just vanish once you're grown up. It sticks around and seeps into how you act and feel every day. And this pain? It doesn't stay put. It travels through the family tree, touching everyone.

Family trauma affects how you see each other. Maybe **trust** has become a rarity. Maybe silence feels safer than speaking up. Imagine trying to bond with people who think you might hurt them or who don't trust your motives. It makes life, even the simple parts, feel like climbing an endless mountain.

But why does this keep happening? Well, trauma can sneak its way down through the generations. Families have weird but strong ways of holding onto rough stuff. This trauma doesn't appear out of nowhere—constant exposure to harm or hurt starts patterns. These behaviors, these ways of thinking, can stick around as long as the family does. Think about a grandfather who saw everything as a threat, yelled often, and never gave enough affection. Those behaviors might teach kids that life is scary and people are the enemy. Then those kids grow up keeping these ideas and might even act them out with their own kids.

When trauma isn't fixed, it trickles into every part of your life. It digs its claws into your **relationships**. You're standing there wanting trust and closeness, but your brain's yelling, "Be careful, you'll get hurt!" Suddenly, it's super hard to feel safe or happy with people. So relationships suffer, often collapsing even though you want them to stay strong.

Personal **growth** is another victim. Maybe you want to better yourself, try new things, but there's a part of you that keeps whispering incomprehensible fears. These stuck feelings from the past tie you down, making change or self-improvement feel terrifying or impossible.

Let's imagine you with unresolved trauma—maybe your self-worth took a hit early on. Relationships could bring out obsessive neediness or complete emotional walled gardens. Or, in work and personal achievements, self-sabotage becomes the norm. "I'll mess up anyway," seems to drown all motivation.

By looking at family trauma closely, it's clear just how much it creeps into every corner of life. Facing these roots and breaking the **cycle** gives hope for happier futures, stronger bonds, and a self that's no longer weighed down. So, understanding and addressing family trauma is really the starting line to freeing yourself and moving forward.

Talking about family trauma helps open up ways to fix it. Knowing you're stuck is the first step to getting unstuck. When you peel away the layers and understand how these patterns formed, it becomes easier to let go. So, it's crucial—beyond crucial, actually—for you to work on this, even if it's tough going at it bit by bit. With time and **effort**, yeah, you can **heal**.

Recognizing Signs of Inherited Trauma

Alright, let's dig into how inherited trauma shows up. You've got them—those **emotional**, behavioral, and physical signs that pop up, but sometimes they're more than just your own stuff.

You might feel **anxiety** out of nowhere or have trouble trusting others even when there's no reason not to. It's like you're carrying someone else's emotional baggage. **Depression** can hit hard too and stick around with feelings of hopelessness that don't quite make sense in the context of your own life. You might also find yourself lashing out in anger, or feeling overly responsible for family members. These are telltale emotional signs that family trauma has taken root in you.

Behavior-wise, inherited trauma can look like avoiding certain situations that remind you of family dramas you never even witnessed yourself. Ever notice patterns of **addiction** or self-destructive habits in family stories? Whether it's substance abuse or just plain old self-sabotage, these behaviors often pass from one generation to the next. Unhealthy relationship patterns can chase you too, sometimes making you repeat the same mistakes over and over.

The physical side of things can be baffling. Chronic pain, headaches, or stomach issues pop up with no clear medical cause. Your body is like a storage unit for that old, unresolved stress. Always tired, even when you sleep a lot? That could be inherited trauma messing with your body's natural rhythms.

Now, let's talk about "**emotional echoes**." These are those ghostly aftereffects of trauma that didn't start with you. Emotional echoes are signals sent out by unresolved stuff from past generations. Say your grandparent went through severe hardship; even if it didn't happen to you directly, you might still feel a reverberation of their grief or anxiety.

These echoes often manifest as those same emotional issues we just went over. Imagine feeling an overwhelming sense of fear in certain situations without knowing why. That's an emotional echo—like you're hearing whispers of a trauma that someone else in your family lived through. Emotional echoes are kind of eerie, right? But spotting them can actually help you disrupt that loop.

To really get a handle on inherited trauma, you've got to look for repeating **patterns** and themes. Sit down and think about any recurring issues within your family. Do several people struggle with the same types of mental health issues? Is there a pattern of broken relationships or unemotional parenting styles?

Check out family histories for repetitive behaviors. Even patterns that seem unrelated might connect once you dig a little deeper. Keep an eye on how your own issues align with these family stories. For example, if frustration around authority is a common thread, you might realize that's been passed down generation to generation.

Once you start spotting these patterns, it's like you're solving a puzzle. And figuring out where your pieces fit can be life-changing. Knowing that your struggles aren't just your own can unburden you a bit. Because it isn't all on you—you're part of a link in the chain.

So, catching these signs, from emotional echoes to repeating patterns, makes you more **aware**. Being aware lets you begin to **heal**—not just yourself, but the ripple effects through past and future generations.

Recognize these signs, tune in to those echoes, and map those patterns. And in getting this better understanding, you're already taking steps toward healing inherited family trauma. You'll start feeling lighter, bit by bit. See? It is possible to rewrite your personal story, and in turn, aim for a more positive future.

The Impact on Personal Well-being

Have you ever **pondered** how trauma gets passed down the family line, like an unwanted heirloom? It's wild how family traumas can sneak into your life and shape who you become. Take **mental health**, for instance. Anxiety and depression often have roots in these deep-seated issues. Imagine growing up in a household full of suppressed emotions, conflicts, or unspoken wounds. These situations embed themselves in your psyche, and you might find yourself dealing with anxiety that seems to come out of nowhere.

It's not just about worrying over your own stuff, but also carrying the weight of what your parents and grandparents went through. It feels like everyone's **nightmares** got packed into a little box and handed down to you. This accumulation of emotional baggage can sneakily creep into your daily life, making ordinary moments more stressful and frazzling. And yeah, it's tough.

But what's even worse? This transferred **trauma** doesn't just stop at making you anxious or sad. It dives into your very identity. Unresolved family trauma can become part of who you are. Your **self-worth** and what you believe makes you "you" can get all tangled up with these old family issues. If your self-esteem takes a hit each time there's a family showdown, or if you're constantly battling to please an emotionally scarred parent, you might start thinking there's something inherently wrong with you. It's not even about who you are right now – it's about inherited fears and doubts.

These past traumas affect your **choices** too. You might find yourself choosing a path just to avoid triggering certain family dynamics. Maybe you don't pick a career you're passionate about because it clashes with what's expected. Or think about the relationships you're in. If your family had toxic dynamics or unresolved conflicts, you might unconsciously seek similar scenarios, just because that's what feels familiar – messed up, right?

Speaking of **relationships**, have you heard of "trauma bonding"? It's a term that gives deep insight into why you sometimes stay in unhealthy connections. When you've grown up witnessing or experiencing trauma, your lines defining love and harm blur. Trauma bonding happens when you form emotional attachments with people who hurt you because, weirdly enough, their behavior mimics the caretakers or family members you once (or still) crave validation from.

So, you meet someone, and their unpredictable or harmful behavior triggers a kind of emotional reflex. You stick around because somewhere inside, reconciling with them feels like winning over a parent's affection you never had. It sounds irrational, but it's rooted in that old hurt.

And it's not just romantic relationships where this plays out. Think of how you manage **boundaries** at work or with friends. Boundaries are meant to protect you, but when you're used to your limits not being respected, you might not set them properly. Or maybe you let people overstep, mistaking invasion for connection. It's a cascade of old learned habits playing out over and over.

So yeah, it's incredible (and not in the good way) how unresolved family trauma can rain down like this persistent drizzle that never quite goes away. Anxiety, depression, splintered identities, poor choices, messed up relationships – all wrapped up in a not-so-neat package handed to you by your lineage. Understanding these threads is rough but essential to untangling them and starting to heal.

Breaking the Cycle of Generational Wounds

Ever feel like you're trapped in a loop, replaying the same painful scenes your family did back in the day? Like you're carrying some invisible bag filled with stuff. **Trauma-informed healing** could be your ticket out of this cycle. It's not just about talking in therapy. It starts with knowing how past traumas affect you now. It's like getting a manual for life's trickiest parts. And guess what? When you understand this stuff, you're already halfway to healing.

So, what's trauma-informed healing anyway? It's about understanding that your actions, thoughts, and feelings are shaped by past experiences. Some of these experiences aren't even yours – they belong to the family before you. Recognizing this makes you less hard on yourself and others. It stops that ugly blame game. You begin to treat yourself with the kindness you never knew you needed. **Healing** doesn't just stick a Band-Aid on the wound; it changes the way you think and react, breaking that old cycle for good.

But knowing's not enough, right? You also gotta tweak the way you deal with life daily. This is where being **self-aware** and making conscious choices comes in. Being aware of your inherited emotional baggage helps you make better decisions. Decisions that don't lead to repeating past mistakes. When you wake up every day, asking how your past affects today, you're already shifting the balance.

Every time you choose to act differently than your default reactions, you're writing a new story. It takes small daily **choices**. Like, deciding to talk to your partner instead of shutting down. Or choosing to breathe deeply instead of yelling when you feel stressed. These actions, as tiny as they seem, free you from past patterns. You're reclaiming your power, one choice at a time.

Alright, so here you are, aware of your past, making better daily choices. What's next? Re-scripting family **stories**. Sounds fancy, huh? It's simpler than it sounds. It's about changing the narrative that's been told for generations and giving it a healthier twist. Think of it this way: your grandparent might have had a tough time, and that hardship got passed down as a sort of gloomy family myth. You can start to edit this. Where there were only tales of suffering, you bring in stories of strength and **resilience**.

You can say, "Yeah, life was hard for them, but they also showed incredible courage." This shift can change everything. When you start seeing the past through a lens of growth and resilience, it affects how you see yourself too. You're no longer a victim of past trauma, but part of a lineage of **survivors**. It's empowering. Every time you share these re-scripted stories, you help yourself and others heal. You're not erasing the old story; you're enriching it.

Rewriting family narratives also invites others to see possibilities beyond the pains they're used to. It gives your family a fresh **identity**, one built on strength and love instead of just tragedy.

All these steps, understanding trauma, making conscious choices, and re-scripting family stories come together in a harmonious way to break the generational cycle. By taking these steps, you help free not just yourself, but also those who come after you. Sounds pretty good, right?

In Conclusion

In this chapter, you've uncovered some **vital truths** about the nature of family trauma and its impact on your life. Understanding these concepts can help you begin the **healing process** and improve your well-being. By becoming aware of your own family history and learning how to address inherited issues, you can create a more **positive future** for yourself and your family.

You've seen what family trauma is and how it affects individual and family well-being. You've learned how trauma can be passed down through generations via behaviors, beliefs, and emotions. You've discovered how **hidden family trauma** can show up in different aspects of life such as relationships and personal growth. You've also learned about signs of family trauma, which can include certain emotional, behavioral, and physical traits. Finally, you've understood the importance of recognizing and breaking the cycle of **generational trauma** for a healthier life.

Let this chapter inspire you to take the steps needed to understand and heal from your family's past. Applying what you've learned can lead to more **fulfilling relationships** and personal growth. Everyone has the power to break the chain of trauma. So why not start this **journey toward healing** today? You've got this, man! It's time to take charge and create the life you deserve. Remember, it's not about blaming anyone; it's about understanding and moving forward. Let's kick off this transformation together!

Chapter 2: The Science Behind Inherited Trauma

Ever wondered how the past can somehow shape your present? I used to ponder that too. Like, can an experience you never had really **affect** you? Guess what - you're in for a revelation.

This chapter will immerse you in strange yet fascinating **theories**. You're about to uncover secrets lying deep within you, ready to reshape how you see your own **feelings** and reactions. Yeah, this goes beyond simple self-help. Ever felt you're reliving someone else's **stress**? Here you'll find out why!

I believe the magic lies in realizing how much our past affects today. So, flip the page. **Dive** in. What you'll learn here might just make you nod and say, "Ah, that makes sense."

Ready? Let's go on this **adventure** together into the hidden depths of **trauma**, waiting for you to **unravel**...

Epigenetics and Trauma Transmission

Let's dive into something pretty **fascinating** but also a bit complex – epigenetics. It's all about how environmental influences can affect gene activity without changing your DNA sequence. Imagine your genes are like piano keys, always there, always the same. Epigenetics is like the piano player, deciding which keys to hit and which ones to avoid. It doesn't alter the piano itself, but it can totally change the tune. This is how traits, and even **trauma**, can be handed down from one generation to the next.

What's really eye-opening is understanding that trauma isn't just in your mind but can have physical imprints on you. Historical trauma, like war, famine, or abuse, doesn't just vanish – it leaves marks. Studies have shown that the experiences of your parents and grandparents can affect you. These traumatic experiences might tweak the expression of certain genes, turning some on or off. This means you might be carrying stress or anxiety simply because your ancestors lived through tough times.

Imagine growing up in a war zone. The constant stress and danger can activate or silence specific genes in the brain linked to stress responses. These changes might get passed on to the next generation through germ cells – meaning your kids could have heightened stress responses even if they grow up in a peaceful environment. Isn't that something?

Now, let's talk about how your **environment** changes gene activity. Every day, you're exposed to various factors like diet, stress, toxins, and even social interactions. These factors can affect which genes are turned on or off. If you're eating healthier, your "good" genes might get activated, promoting better health. Or, if you're constantly under stress, it might activate genes tied to inflammation or stress hormones. The kicker? These changes don't usually alter your DNA. Instead, they modify the "epigenetic markers," which are sort of tags on your DNA that influence gene activity.

Think about identical twins growing up in different environments – one in a nurturing home, the other in a volatile one. Even though their DNA is identical, their epigenetic markers will be different, affecting their health and psyche. Scientists are learning more about this and finding that these tags are not sealed forever. They're kind of like sticky notes that can be placed, removed, or shifted around under different circumstances.

Recent research is shining a light on trauma's epigenetic effects across **generations**. In one study, children of Holocaust survivors exhibited changes in the FKBP5 gene, which is involved in stress regulation. Though these children didn't experience the traumatic events themselves, their stress responses were evidently shaped by the traumas their parents went through.

Another fascinating study focused on mice. Researchers found that exposing pregnant mice to stress changed the behavior and brain chemistry of their offspring. These offspring showed increased symptoms of anxiety and depression, and what's even crazier, this continued for multiple generations. It wasn't just a fluke; something real changed in their genes or, well, in their markers.

What does this mean for you? It confirms how deeply experiences can shape individuals and stretch across generations. This knowledge can **empower** you to make informed choices about lifestyle and mental health. The idea that traumas can be inherited may sound a bit grim, but it also opens doors to healing. If negative experiences can pass down, so can positive interventions – like mindfulness, a supportive environment, or therapies, potentially rewriting those epigenetic tags for the better.

In essence, epigenetics is like a bridge connecting your environment with your genes, affecting you and possibly future generations. And this is why understanding it matters, especially when it comes to healing from family **trauma**. It gives you insights and tools to break the cycle, to ensure that the melody your piano plays for your future generations is one of **resilience** and **strength**.

Neurobiological Effects of Family Trauma

Understanding how **trauma** changes the brain might seem overwhelming, but stick with me. We're talking about real physical changes here. Family trauma doesn't just mess with your head emotionally—there are actual changes to your brain's structure and function.

Take the parts of the brain tied to emotion control and **memory**, like the amygdala and hippocampus. Your amygdala, often called the brain's smoke alarm, can get hyperactive. That means it goes off at the slightest hint of danger, even when there isn't any real threat. Meanwhile, your hippocampus—crucial for creating new memories—can shrink. This can make it tough to remember new facts or focus on what's happening right now because it's too busy freaking out about past hurts.

Now, here comes the hopeful bit. **Brain plasticity**, or how your brain can change and adapt. This means those changes trauma causes aren't set in stone. Think of your brain like a forest—the paths (neural connections) get used over and over again, becoming well-trodden but avoiding others. If the forest has pathways created from trauma, it doesn't mean they're permanent. New paths can form with the right experiences and efforts.

Recovery from trauma taps into brain plasticity. Activities like mindfulness and therapy work like a gardening hoe, helping you carve out new routes. The more you use these new paths, the more natural they become, until the old, negative responses fall out of disuse.

But how does this horror story of hand-me-down trauma even happen? Enter the **limbic system**, your brain's emotional hub. Think of it as the ancient, deep-set part of your brain tasked with survival. When something traumatic happens, the limbic system doesn't just note it; it takes it in, absorbs it, holds onto it. It's always on alert.

Memory-wise, it's like keeping a family photo album, but instead of pictures, it's filled with emotional feedback from past experiences. This album can get passed down generation to generation. So, if your ancestors experienced trauma, their survival responses might get hardwired into your brain, making you more sensitive or reactive to **stress**. Almost like inheriting your mom's eyes but way less fun.

Combining all these thoughts—the changed brain structures, the power of brain plasticity, and the role of the limbic system—gives you a fuller picture of family trauma. It changes your brain, rearranges the paths you walk daily, but also offers **hope** with the ability you have to create new, healthier paths.

In sum, the brain isn't a rigid command center but more of a flexible workspace. Even though trauma reshapes emotional regulation and memory, it's entirely possible to rebuild. With time, patience, and sometimes a good therapist's help, you can alter those ingrained responses.

In my opinion, knowing this offers profound **peace**. Your brain can heal, and recovery is well within reach.

Stress Responses and Inherited Patterns

You know how sometimes your **reactions** to stress seem more like automatic buttons than thoughtful choices? That's because you have what's called "adaptive stress responses." Over time, though, these can turn unhelpful. For example, when you're a kid living in a house that feels unsafe, you might get really good at being alert all the time, watching for danger. At that moment, it might help you **survive**. But as you grow, that constant state of alertness starts to wear you down. Your body can't tell the difference between an actual threat and things like daily work stress or a phone call from your boss.

Your **brain** is like a fire alarm that now goes off whenever there's burnt toast. Those old responses, once helpful, become harmful and exhausting. You might find yourself overreacting to small things, lashing out at loved ones, or just feeling worn out all the time. It's like carrying an emergency siren in your head.

Moving on from old adaptive stress responses, let's talk about passed-down **trauma**. Trauma that affects your parents or grandparents can actually change the way your brain and body respond to stress. It's called inherited or intergenerational trauma. This isn't just about stories your family tells or values they pass down—it's actually in your genetics. When a parent lives through something traumatic, it can literally be written into their DNA. This evolved DNA can make you more sensitive to stress.

Imagine your nervous system being predestined to be more reactive because of what your parents or even grandparents experienced. Maybe your grandparent lived through a war or a famine. That intense stress adjusted their body and brain, and these adjustments get passed down. So you might find you're more jumpy or anxious, even if your own life hasn't had such severe hardships. It's like inheriting an aching back but for your emotional state. That extra **sensitivity** can mess with your daily life, making even minor stress feel overwhelming.

Now, let's look at the health issues intertwined with inherited trauma. When your nervous system is always on high alert, it doesn't just mess with your head—it can mess with your whole body, too. You may have higher cortisol levels all the time, which is the stress **hormone**. This can lead to ongoing health problems like high blood pressure, heart issues, or even digestive problems.

Think about it like this: your body's operating system is stuck in overdrive mode. This means chronic headaches, difficulty sleeping well, or even weaker immune response - constantly catching colds or feeling under the weather. Inherited trauma plants the seed, and everyday stress waters it into a full-blown health issue. Sometimes, the health problems feel like they're out of nowhere, but they may be deeply rooted in your family lines.

Understanding these connections gives you the tools to tackle stress and trauma head-on. If you recognize how these patterns form, tracing them back to inherited roots, you can start finding ways to break the **cycle**. When you work through this inherited baggage, you grant yourself the chance to create a healthier, more balanced **future**.

The Role of the Autonomic Nervous System

Alright, let's talk about the autonomic nervous system. This bad boy is like your body's **autopilot**. Most of the stuff it does, you don't even have to think about. It's always running the show in the background. Think heartbeats, digestion, and even that slight sweat when you're a bit nervous. The autonomic nervous system has two main parts: the **sympathetic** and **parasympathetic** branches.

The sympathetic branch is like your little warrior or, if you will, the part of you that's always ready for action. When something stressful happens, this is what kicks in. Your heart pounds faster, senses get sharper—basically, you're ready to fight, run, or do whatever's needed in a pinch. On the other side, there's the parasympathetic branch. Let's call this your inner chill mode. It's the calming buddy that helps you relax and brings everything back to a state of peace. Imagine digesting food, resting, or just feeling at ease—that's the parasympathetic doing its thing.

But here's the kicker. **Trauma** messes up this balance big time. When you go through something traumatic, it can tug on the reins of this system and yank them out of alignment. Instead of flowing smoothly between action and rest, you might get stuck in survival mode. And it doesn't just go away when the event is over. The sympathetic branch can stay revved up, always on the lookout for the next threat. This constant state of alert keeps your body on edge and overly stressed, which leaves you dealing with all kinds of problems, both physical and emotional.

So how does this chaos move from one generation to another? Through something called "**neuroception**." Basically, it's how your body senses and responds to safety or danger without you being consciously aware of it. It's like having a built-in radar, constantly scanning the environment for cues. When trauma gets woven into this radar, weird things start happening. Small triggers can set off big reactions because this altered system is always sensing a threat, even when there isn't one.

And here's the wild part—this gets inherited. Your radar doesn't reset with each new family member. Those trauma responses get passed down. Kids learn from their parents without even knowing it, embedding those fears and **triggers** deep inside. Your body might respond to stresses in ways that feel ancient, because, in a way, they are. Generational trauma means parts of you react as though they're living in past horrors—sometimes without you even realizing why.

Okay, I know it sounds intense but understanding this is half the battle. You have this complex system, messed up by trauma, and perpetuating a cycle of hyper-vigilance and unneeded stress responses through neuroception. But knowing this is empowering because when you're aware of the autonomic nervous system's role, you start recognizing those misleading danger signals. That's a start towards resetting the balance, not just for yourself, but potentially for future **generations** too.

Got it? Good. This groundwork makes it easier to figure out healing steps and ultimately create more peace within yourself and your family lineage.

In Conclusion

In this chapter, you've learned about the **science** behind inherited **trauma** and how it impacts you. Understanding these concepts can help you make sense of your own **feelings** and those of your family. Remember, you have the power to begin **healing** from past hurts.

Throughout this chapter, you've explored what epigenetics is and how it connects with **trauma** passed down from parent to child. You've discovered that environmental influences can change how **genes** behave without messing with the DNA itself. Recent studies have shown how trauma affects generations through epigenetics, and you've learned how family trauma changes the **brain**, especially areas tied to emotions and **memories**.

You've also gained insight into the nervous system's role in trauma and why balancing it is essential to prevent stress-related issues. Keep these points in mind as you consider the power you hold to start healing from family trauma. Make each day count towards understanding more, healing more, and creating a brighter future for yourself and those around you.

Chapter 3: Identifying Your Family Trauma Patterns

Ever **wondered** why you react a certain way? Does it feel like **history** from generations ago somehow echoes in your daily life? In this chapter, you'll begin a **journey** that might just shake the way you view yourself and your place within your family. I've been where you are - perplexed by the emotional currents that seem to invisibly steer my actions. Recognizing those unseen **patterns** and emotional inheritances is the initial step.

You might **discover** hidden stories that have been kept in the shadows or overlooked whispers that hold the key to understanding your struggles today. Together, we'll **map** out your family's emotional legacy, connecting today's challenges with events from the past. This might seem daunting, but it's an eye-opener that'll shift your **perspective** dramatically.

Diving into this chapter, you're about to uncover what's been beneath the surface. It's time to peel back the layers and get to the root of those family **trauma** patterns. Trust me, it's a game-changer. You'll start seeing connections you never noticed before, and it might just explain a lot about why you do what you do.

So, buckle up and get ready for some serious self-discovery. This isn't just about digging up old family dirt; it's about understanding yourself better and maybe even breaking some cycles that have been running on repeat for generations. It's heavy stuff, but don't worry -

we're in this together, and by the end, you'll have a whole new toolkit for dealing with your family's emotional baggage.

Recognizing Emotional Inheritance

What is emotional inheritance anyway? It's like carrying invisible **baggage** handed down through generations. You might not realize it, but the way you **react** to certain situations and your emotional responses can be influenced by what your ancestors felt and experienced. Imagine emotional patterns passed down like family heirlooms, only they aren't pieces of jewelry or old letters. They're **feelings**, instincts, ways of dealing—or not dealing—with problems.

Often, you don't question why you feel nervous as soon as something goes slightly wrong or why sadness sometimes seeps in for no apparent reason. These may be signs of emotional inheritance. Maybe your grandmother was always anxious, jumpy, worrying over every little thing. Without knowing it, that energetic bundle of anxiety could've been handed down to you. It's not your fault; it's just **genes** mixed with experiences that shape your everyday behavior.

Thinking deeper, notice these common emotional habits as hints of inherited **trauma**. Always feeling edgy or worried when there's nothing really wrong? There could be past family tensions bubbling under the surface. What about those days when you can't pinpoint why you're sad, yet the emotion feels so heavy? These can be subtle signals of emotional inheritance working its mischief. They whisper that something from the past still lingers.

Switching gears a bit, family emotional **atmosphere** is super important too. Think about the emotional climate growing up in your family's home. Was it filled with tension, unspoken grudges, or unexpressed love? If your parents or caregivers habitually dealt with stress by shutting down or lashing out, you likely picked up on these cues. Maybe your dad bottled everything inside, never spilled a tear, and now you find it hard to cry even when you want to. This is how the family emotional atmosphere shapes your every reaction and stress-handling mechanism.

Life's pressures aren't new, but how each family deals with them varies. Imagine **stress** as a leaky faucet. Some families run around patching it up calmly, while others might blow a fuse. How did your family handle that drip-drip-drip? Calmly addressing it or panicking about the flood? And guess what? You probably handle stress the same way. Your emotional responses are influenced by what you saw back home.

In my opinion, taking a closer look at what's been passed down helps to free yourself from these patterns. It's like when you know a spooky tale isn't real, it's not as scary anymore. Same goes for family trauma patterns; understand them, and you can take control over them.

Wrapping all this up, getting to know your emotional baggage sourced from your family can change the game. It doesn't vanish overnight, but each step of **recognition** paves the way to feel lighter and better equipped for the future. You might find yourself reacting differently, making deliberate choices for you and the emotional fingerprints you leave behind, and creating a space where stress is handled with more care and less inherited reaction.

So, take a deep breath. Look back so you can choose how you want to feel moving forward. After all, knowing your emotional inheritance isn't just about understanding the past—it's about shaping your emotional **future** too.

Uncovering Family Secrets and Silences

Ever notice how family reunions sometimes feel a bit awkward? It's not just because of the small talk or long-lost second cousins. Many families have buried **secrets**. Stuff you don't talk about. The unspoken **traumas** that go hush-hush often leave scars that last for generations. Not on the skin, though. On the soul.

For many, uncovering these hidden traumas is like opening Pandora's box. It's daunting, sometimes even terrifying. These secrets are often tied up with shame, fear, or a desire to protect someone. But when these wounds stay hidden, they fester. They can affect your **relationships**, your sense of self, and even your dreams. Imagine carrying a bag that's not even yours—and it's filled with stuff you didn't pack.

Okay, take a second to pardon the gloominess here. The real deal is, while origins of the trauma come from back in the day, the effects are very present today. Whether it's an old feud nobody talks about or a tragic event everyone pretends never happened, these secrets act like invisible threads, pulling everyone along, subconsciously. But realizing that the cause of your own personal struggles stems from family stories helps you shift—find some relief. It's like connecting pieces of a bigger puzzle.

But isn't ignoring these secrets easier? That brings us to the concept of a "conspiracy of **silence**." Think of it like this unspoken agreement that everyone knows but nobody admits to. When a family collectively decides to keep secrets buried, they create more silence. This silence acts like dense fog, making it tough for anyone to find clarity or **healing**. It builds walls between people, locks hearts in cages, keeps painful mysteries unsolved.

Here's the thing—toothaches don't heal by themselves, do they? Similarly, silence won't fix trauma. This conspiracy drags down generations like an anchor, and often, you don't even notice until you confront it. Over and over, it keeps generations stuck in toxic patterns. The avoidance, the sniff of dread each time the subject comes close—they just perpetuate the cycle.

Breaking this silence is a hard yet necessary boss battle. By encouraging open chat about true family **history**, you lessen the fog. The dialogue doesn't bring up only problems but solutions. It opens windows to rooms locked forever. Sure, it means opening up a past that many would've preferred staying shut. But the openness fosters understanding and connection. It bridges the gap between the past and present, blending old scars with new hopes.

Actually talking about these hard memories—this is where healing sneaks in. No need for those deep-your-heart discussions if it feels too raw. Start small. Maybe a tale at dinner. A chat in the car. Little dots along the way help create a whole picture. This habit-breaking stirs a whole mix of emotions for everyone involved—fear, hope, anger, maybe even peace—but it ensures wounds get aired out.

Transitioning into talking about these matters initially can be tough. You might feel nervous. Probably worried how relatives will react. But soon, as if miraculously, speaking freely becomes the norm, not avoiding topics. Suddenly, healing your story regarding the bloom—it sets the foundation to breathe easy and have healthy **communication**.

Family history casts a shadow. But denying shadows won't make it sunny. Addressing these buried issues lays the groundwork for a healthier, happier future. No guilt in looking back, questioning, understanding. By embracing—or facing—the narratives past generations imparted, you sort of disrupt the toxic pattern for **generations** yet to come.

Tangled up in layers of humor and scars are stories wishing to find a voice, secrets wanting to breathe fresh air. From dancing around it, brushing it under the rug, to courageously connecting dots and making sense of them. It's an effort synonymous with removing cactus needles, coupled with this powerful reality: looking backward genuinely makes the way forward brighter.

Mapping Your Family's Emotional Legacy

Think about an emotional genogram like a family tree, but way **cooler**. Instead of just focusing on who's who, it digs into your family's emotional history—kinda like playing **detective** with your feelings. You get to see **patterns** and behaviors that run deep, often across several generations. So, how do you make this all work?

Start with pen and paper or one of those apps if you prefer. Draw a simple tree structure: you, your siblings, parents, grandparents, and so on. But don't just stick to the basics. Add **relationships**, emotions, and key life events like divorces, illnesses, or even financial troubles. Notice how these events impacted emotions and behaviors. Maybe your grandpa was distant because he lost his wife young. Or your mom is anxious because her mom was always fretting about money.

Now, pay attention to recurring themes. Are there patterns of anger, sadness, or even joy? Sure, spotting these can feel a bit heavy, but it's powerful stuff. You might find that a sense of abandonment shows up in every generation. Or there might be a pattern of perfectionism or being overly critical. These themes help you understand why certain traits stick around like that stubborn stain on your favorite T-shirt.

Understanding these patterns is your ticket to breaking the **cycle**. It's not about blaming anyone but about recognizing why things are as they are. Once you've noticed these trends, it becomes easier to change your own story. You're wiser now, you've got information, and information is power. So take that knowledge and make intentional changes, ensuring the emotional baggage stops with you.

Alright, you've got your family map and patterns spotted. But what's buried beneath those patterns? Enter the process of emotional **archaeology**. That's like digging beneath the surface to uncover hidden family traumas. These are often the buried stories that folks don't talk about, yet they continue to haunt generation after generation.

Start by asking questions and having real conversations. Talk to your parents, grandparents—whoever will listen. Ask them about their struggles, their pain points. You'll be surprised how much gets swept under the rug, gathering dust, yet impacting everyone. Sometimes just having open, honest communication about these hidden traumas brings a sense of understanding and even healing.

You might also need to look at societal or historical events that impacted your family. Maybe your family went through war, economic hardships, or social upheaval. These big events can leave emotional scars that are passed down, even if no one directly talks about them. It's as if they imprint on the family's emotional DNA, influencing reactions and behaviors.

But it doesn't end there. This digging will unveil the impacts these traumas have on your family's behaviors and emotions. Once you're aware of these traumas and their rippling effects, you've got more pieces to your personal puzzle. It helps explain why certain reactions and behaviors get "inherited," so to speak, without anyone really realizing it.

So, why does this matter? Well, knowing the "why" behind your family's emotional legacy gives you the kind of insight that can guide your **healing** journey. You'll start seeing emotional patterns not as personal failures but as inherited tales waiting to be rewritten.

By using emotional genograms, uncovering patterns, and diving into emotional archaeology, you're setting yourself up to better understand and, most importantly, to heal. So rise above the noise of the past trauma, clear out the emotional clutter, and create that positive future you've been longing for. It's entirely possible, and you've got the tools in hand to start today.

Connecting Present Struggles to Past Events

Ever feel like the past is creeping into your present? **Trauma** does that. It might make old events feel like they're happening right now, coloring your everyday life. Imagine you're getting worked up about something small, only to realize it's not just about the present moment. It's as if that old wound never really healed and is still throbbing.

These blasts from the past can mess with your day-to-day. You might find yourself **overreacting** to stuff that shouldn't bother you so much. It's weird how you can be fine one minute and spiraling the next. It's like you're living in a loop where past and present blur into one big mess.

Recognizing these emotional echoes in your life is key to making sense of things. Start by paying attention to recurring **patterns**. Is there a particular situation that always stirs up strong feelings? Those are clues pointing straight back to old family traumas. It's like shining a light on stuff hiding in your blind spot.

If every disagreement with a loved one feels like the end of the world, there's probably an old scar involved. Emotional echoes don't come out of nowhere. They repeat the pain we've seen or felt before, often passed down through generations. It's tricky, too, because it can be subtle. You might not even notice these echoes at first, but they're there, haunting you and shaping your reactions.

Now, why connect your personal **struggles** to your family's history? Because seeing the bigger picture helps more than you'd think. When you realize that your anxiety during family gatherings isn't just your problem but a shadow from your grandparent's turbulent past, it hits different. You're not alone in this. That pressure to be perfect might come from a legacy of unmet expectations, passed down like unwanted heirlooms.

Placing your struggles in **context** doesn't just give you perspective; it offers a kind of validation. Your battles aren't random, they're rooted in a deeper context. And that context? It shapes who you are, even if you're unaware of it. Sometimes it helps to map this out—literally. Draw a family tree and note conflicts, patterns, or even recurrent mental health issues to reveal connections you didn't see before.

Understanding these links between past and present gives you a grip on things. It doesn't make everything okay, but it does provide a **roadmap**. You start seeing when an issue is yours and when it's something inherited. When those emotional echoes start to scream, you can say, "Oh, this feels familiar—maybe it's something more."

So, when dealing with your own struggles, take a step back. Think about where they might really come from. Looking into your family's past can be like peeling back layers on an onion. Each layer brings its own set of tears, but it gets you closer to the core of what's driving your **emotions** today. Understanding this, in my opinion, can help you start **healing**, freeing you bit by bit from the emotional baggage of the past.

In Conclusion

In this chapter, you've **explored** the impact of family trauma on your emotions and behavior. It's crucial to delve into these patterns to **understand** and heal from them. By recognizing emotional inheritance and uncovering hidden family secrets, you can begin to **address** the emotional wounds that persist across generations. This understanding allows you to live a healthier and more fulfilling life.

You've seen how "emotional inheritance" **shapes** your responses to life events. You've learned to spot patterns indicating inherited trauma, like chronic anxiety or sudden sadness. You've discovered the effects of family secrets on multiple generations and the role of "conspiracy of silence" in keeping hidden traumas alive. You've also been introduced to tools like "emotional genograms" to visualize and **decode** family emotional patterns.

Take these lessons to heart. By acknowledging these patterns and working towards understanding them, you can **break** the cycle of inherited trauma. Remember, the path to emotional freedom starts with awareness and openness. Keep **striving** to understand and heal, and you can create a more positive future for yourself and your family.

Chapter 4: The Language of Inherited Trauma

Ever felt like you're carrying the **weight** of emotions that aren't exactly yours? Well, I know I have. This chapter is your **guide** to decode and make sense of those feelings. We'll dive into your core emotional **vocabulary** together, identifying recurring **themes** that keep popping up in your life. Ready to uncover some hidden family **stories** and beliefs you didn't even know you had? It's going to be quite a journey.

You see, understanding these ingrained **patterns** can truly change the way you look at yourself. As you read, you'll get to piece together parts of your emotional **puzzle**. Don't we all want to understand why we think and act the way we do? By the time you're done with this chapter, you'll start seeing those puzzle pieces fall perfectly into place. Dive in; there's a lot to **discover** about what makes you, well, you.

Decoding Your Core Emotional Vocabulary

Have you ever noticed how certain **feelings** keep popping up in your life, almost like uninvited guests? You're dealing with sadness, grief, or maybe anger that seems to come out of nowhere. What's interesting is, these might be hinting at something deeper. See, recurring emotional themes could be whispers of **inherited trauma**. Stuff your parents dealt with, maybe even their parents before them.

It's like running into the same emotional walls without knowing where they came from.

Picture this: You're having a great day, and suddenly, a random comment throws you into a pit of sadness. Maybe that's not just "you." It's like leftovers from someone else's emotional meal. These recurring feelings are kind of your emotional **fingerprints**. Unique quirks tracing back to what your parents or grandparents might have experienced. **Emotion** tends to stick around, passing from one generation to the next, subtle yet powerful. These patterns aren't just yours—they belong to your family tree.

Let's chew on this "emotional fingerprint" idea a bit more. Think of them as invisible marks left by family **trauma** patterns. Like how some families pass down heirlooms, others unintentionally pass down emotional states. Often, you're walking around burdened by someone else's baggage. These emotional fingerprints are sneaky. You might snap at someone for no real reason or feel deep sadness out of the blue. Those fingerprints are there to remind you your ancestors have been through stuff, and you've picked up their emotional breadcrumbs.

So, how might you track these elusive emotions in your life? Let's talk about emotion **mapping**. Grab a pen or maybe open a doc on your computer. List out your most common emotions. Sadness, anger, anxiety—whatever features most in your life. Now, think about your day-to-day situations. Who are you with when you feel these emotions? What's going on around you? Jot these down too.

Got your list? Now note the frequency. How often are you feeling this stuff? Is there a pattern? Certain times of the day or situations? Recognizing this helps you see if these feelings are out of place. Let's say every time you talk with your sibling, you feel this overwhelming sadness. That's something worth paying attention to. Patterns like that give clues. And hey, honesty with yourself is crucial here.

Got your patterns in check? Hold tight for an important step. Reflect on them deeply—these recurring emotions tell you where to poke around more. Your sadness might not be just yours; it could link back to how your mom always strained while dealing with loss, or maybe how your granddad fought back tears during family dinners. Tracking this stuff isn't to dwell on sadness but so you start choosing your reactions.

Understanding these clues makes surprising sense once laid out clearly. Your emotional **vocabulary** needs decoding to set a cleaner future. In spotting, fingerprinting, and mapping these themes – congratulations, you're breaking a generational cycle. Whether it's anger or moments of loneliness, these emotions have histories begging for clarity.

So, there you have it. Pay attention to the recurring themes spilling into your daily chores. Track how your family's past shapes who you are today. These small steps help in understanding why certain emotions hit you. And in knowing where they came from, you reclaim your emotional **landscape** – one snapshot, one fingerprint, and one map at a time.

Identifying Recurring Themes in Your Life

Understanding how to spot those repeating life situations is super useful. You know, the kind that makes you feel like you're stuck in a loop. It's not just bad luck or coincidence, most of the time. These patterns often come from **family trauma** that maybe you didn't even know you had. Think about it like this: your family passes down more than just genes, right? They also hand off behaviors, beliefs, and reactions. So, you might keep facing the same issues over and over because of this.

Let's take a closer look at these repeating life situations. Imagine always ending up in the same sort of bad **relationships** or finding yourself feeling unworthy at work. Odds are, these scenarios are connected to past family experiences. Maybe your parents had an unsteady relationship, or there was always tension around money growing up. Now, you're walking in those same footsteps without realizing it.

Here's something interesting. This stuff happens because of something called "**life scripts**." Essentially, life scripts are like pre-written plays, and you're one of the actors following them without even knowing. These scripts get shaped by the traumas passed down through your family. For example, if your grandparents went through tough times, they might've passed on a scarcity mindset. Next thing you know, you're making choices based on the idea that you never have enough, even when you do.

These life scripts are sneaky because they work in the background. You find yourself acting out old stories, even when they don't seem to make much sense today. They shape your reactions and decisions, guiding you toward the same old problems your family faced. And it keeps happening until—well, until you spot them and decide to rewrite them for yourself.

So, how do you do that? One great way is the "**Theme Tracking**" exercise. Grab a notebook or open a new doc on your computer. Start noting down any recurring life patterns you spot. Maybe you always mistrust your partners or never finish what you start. Write those down. Each time it happens, jot down the context. Were you feeling stressed? Was someone else involved? The goal is to identify **triggers** and scenarios.

Once you've got a good list going, set aside some time to review it. Look for common threads. Are people treating you the same way in each situation? Are you reacting the same way each time? The more detailed you are, the better. This helps you see the bigger picture. It helps you realize these patterns aren't random—they're echoes of old scripts.

By the way, don't be too hard on yourself while doing this. Finding these patterns is like peeling an onion—lots of layers, and sometimes it makes you cry a bit. But sticking with it is important because these insights can be really freeing. Spotting these **themes** is a huge step in not repeating them. You get to start making different choices, breaking away from those old scripts.

And that's what it's really about, isn't it? Knowing you've got the power to carve out a new path for yourself. It might take some time and effort, yes, but it's way worth it. Recognizing these patterns and rewriting your life scripts can work wonders for your **emotional well-being**. So go ahead, start that Theme Tracking exercise. You've got nothing to lose except those old, unwanted patterns.

Recognizing Inherited Beliefs and Behaviors

Ever wondered where those persistent **thoughts** in your head come from? Are they truly yours, or did they sneak in from somewhere else? It's fascinating how much of what you believe isn't actually your own creation. Instead, they're hand-me-downs from family, generation after generation. Not always the best gifts, right?

Think about this—you're sitting at home and, out of the blue, you're overly worried about something trivial. Is it really your worry, or could it be something your mom or grandma used to stress about? Unknowingly, you absorb these vibes from family. Like old furniture, they just became part of your household. Your own beliefs and those soaked in from family **trauma** can be hard to separate. One way to tell them apart is to pick them out one by one, and basically ask yourself, "Is this something I chose or something I simply adopted?"

Moving along, let's get into how some coping **methods** get passed down like Grandma's china set. Families have this thing where they handle hardships in a certain style, and that style becomes tradition. Kind of like having a secret family recipe, only it's how to react to stress or pain. Let's say your dad always met problems with anger. So guess what? You might resort to anger when facing a rough patch. Or, if avoiding issues was your family's silent rule, you might find yourself fleeing any conflict. These **behaviors** seep deeply into your character almost as if they were determined even before you had a say in it. Intrigued yet?

But how do you get a grip on what's passed down and fix this chain reaction? Here's where the "Belief Origin" method can help. Picture this as a detective's toolkit. Want to play Sherlock? Start by listing out some of your strongest beliefs and behaviors. Like, "I'm not good enough" or "When things get bad, just flee." List them down. That's clue number one. The next step is about questioning each one. Ask, "When did I first start to feel this?" "Where or who did I get this from?" Try to dig into whether these ideas first formed in your childhood home, maybe rooted in some family story or a parent's reaction. You're trying to recall a moment or an emotional imprint tied to that belief or behavior. It won't always be easy, but dissecting and pinpointing that flashpoint is like shining a flashlight in a hazy room.

Alright, bear with me now—connecting these dots from past to present can be freeing. Once you've tracked down these unwanted guests in your belief house and named them truly as remnants of inherited **trauma**, you get to decide. Do you really want to keep them? Pretty empowering to think you can pack these beliefs back up like unwanted hand-me-downs and leave them behind, huh?

This method isn't a snap-your-fingers fix. But beginning to recognize and label your beliefs and behaviors' **roots** can be a game-changer. Knowing what's yours and what's not gives you the power to reshape your thinking and reactions going forward. So is it your belief or your family's? Unwrapping this **mystery** can lead to more peace and a self that feels genuinely... well, you.

Uncovering Hidden Family Narratives

Sometimes, you might find **unspoken rules** and expectations in your family that don't make sense. It's like there are these invisible strings pulling everyone in certain directions. You might have never given them a second thought, but these strings are often tied to past **traumas**. Families develop these rules to cope with hard times or events that happened long ago. Maybe it's always expected that at family gatherings, nobody talks about certain topics. Or perhaps there's a rule that everyone must put up a strong front, no matter what. It's like walking on eggshells sometimes, isn't it?

Identifying these hidden rules is the first step. Pay attention to things that are off-limits to discuss, or actions that get an over-the-top reaction in a group setting. Notice what things people are allowed to feel or not feel. Do some digging into why these rules might exist. Is there a family story or an old wound that's never healed? Questions lead to more questions, right?

Family **myths** are another way past trauma sticks around. Think of them like bedtime stories passed down with a twist. They don't come with a 'once upon a time', but they do come with a 'because that's just how we do things.' These myths might explain why members of your family always handle things in a certain way. Maybe there's this idea that your family is cursed with bad luck or that you always have to be perfect. Believing these myths keeps you stuck in your tracks, repeating the same old story lines.

These myths give everyone a role they didn't really choose. One person's the caretaker, another's the "black sheep", and so on. Breaking free from these myths means facing up to these roles and shifting them. Easier said than done, right? But understanding this is half the battle.

So, here's how you can start figuring out these hidden stories: through a **Narrative Exploration** exercise. It's not a walk in the park, but it's doable. Grab a pen and some paper, and start asking the right questions. Write down some key family stories you've heard while growing up. Don't be shy - note even the most bizarre ones.

Once you have a list, ask yourself questions about each story. Who told it? Why did they tell it? What's the lesson or rule hidden in it? Dig a bit to uncover the **emotions** that come with these stories. Do they make you feel afraid, proud, or maybe ashamed? These emotions might be the chains of past trauma lurking in your family stories.

Read your notes back to yourself and notice any **patterns**. Are there recurring themes like sacrifice, strength, or any particular fear? Connecting these dots helps in sketching out the puzzle of your family's hidden narrative. It's like becoming a sleuth in your own family history, with your feelings as clues guiding you.

When wrapping things up, remember to be kind to yourself. Digging into family myths can open up some old wounds or create new realizations. It's part of the **healing process**. By spotting those unspoken rules, understanding the myths, and exploring these narratives, you'll start to see where changes are possible. Maybe it unlocks some compassion for that stern uncle, or helps you set a new family rule that heals rather than harms.

And there you go – hidden family narratives are complex but not impossible to uncover. Every story you bring to light is a step towards **healing**. You're piecing together the puzzle and taking control of the narrative. And that's where real change starts.

In Conclusion

In this chapter, we've delved into the **crucial** ways inherited trauma affects you and how you can begin to **understand** and address it. By learning to **recognize** and decode your emotional experiences, you can take the first steps towards **healing** and creating healthier patterns for yourself and your family. Let's sum up the main points to remember.

You've seen how **identifying** recurring emotional themes in your daily life can reveal signs of inherited trauma. We've explored the concept of "emotional fingerprints" that show family trauma patterns. You've learned about the "Emotion Mapping" exercise to **track** and analyze your frequent emotional states. We've also discussed understanding repetitive life situations caused by inherited trauma through "life scripts," and you've discovered the "Theme Tracking" exercise to **identify** common patterns in your life.

As you move forward, remember to **apply** these insights and techniques whenever you feel stuck or overwhelmed by your emotions and life patterns. Your past doesn't have to define your future, and by addressing these deep-rooted issues, you can pave the way for a more positive and fulfilling life.

Keep in mind that this journey of self-discovery and healing is uniquely yours. Don't be too hard on yourself if progress seems slow at times. Every step you take, no matter how small, is moving you in the right direction. Trust the process and be patient with yourself as you navigate these complex emotions and patterns.

Remember, you've got this! With time, effort, and self-compassion, you can break free from the cycle of inherited trauma and create a brighter future for yourself and those around you.

Chapter 5: The Core Language Approach

Ever **wondered** how words can change your life? You're about to find out. In this chapter, I share **methods** that could make you see everything like it's the first time. You'll tackle your own **complaints** so you can figure out what's really bugging you. Then, we get to the heart of the matter, **identifying** key words that help us understand our deepest feelings.

You'll **craft** a sentence that'll capture who you are in a way you've never thought possible. It's a bit like finding your own personal **motto**. We're peeling back layers to reveal the things that've hurt you the most but also define you. There's even a fun way to put it all together – your own language **map** – to navigate your thoughts and understand yourself better.

Ready to **change** how you think and speak? Let's jump in.

Understanding Core Complaints

To start **figuring out** your most persistent life complaints, think about the things that **bug** you regularly. You know, those recurring issues that seem like they're on repeat in your life. These might include conflicts with loved ones, issues at work, or feelings of being unworthy. But here's the twist – these annoyances could be linked to family **trauma**. Think about it like old hand-me-downs. These problems might not even originate from you or your actions.

When you start looking at these frequent gripes, try to see if there's a **pattern**. Are they constant and unchanging? Like, do you always find yourself clashing with authority figures? If yes, it could be something deeper than meets the eye. To get to the root, ask yourself if it's possible that these situations reflect old, inherited wounds.

But how do you tell apart surface-level complaints and deeper core issues? Surface complaints are those fleeting annoyances. Like, being ticked off when you spill coffee on your shirt or missing the bus. But deeper core issues are recurring. They kinda stick with you, popping up again and again in different circumstances.

For instance, if you always feel underappreciated at work, it might link back to feeling ignored as a child. Or constantly fearing failure might trace back to family pressure for excellence. Recognizing these deeper issues involves digging a little further. Don't stop at the obvious. Think about how these patterns might relate to your family **history**.

Alright, so moving on from there, here's a simple trick to help uncover patterns – the "Complaint **Journaling**" technique. Grab a notebook and jot down your daily complaints. Whenever something ruffles your feathers, write it down. But there's more. Write down not just what happened, but also how you felt, and try to trace your feelings back in time.

For example:

• Complaint: Your boss always criticizes your work.

• Feeling: You feel like you're never good enough.

• Connection: This kinda reminds you of how your dad used to nitpick everything you did when you were a kid.

By staying consistent with this journaling practice, you'll start seeing patterns. It's like connecting the dots. You might notice certain phrases that repeat, or feelings that resurface. It's in these patterns that the deeper, inherited trauma might reveal itself. And guess what, just recognizing them can be the first step to **healing**.

In the end, figuring out your core complaints isn't just about whining on paper. It's about diving deep into old wounds and seeing them for what they really are. So next time you find yourself with a persistent problem, grab your journal and take a closer look. You might just be peeling back layers – layers that have been holding you back.

So in summary, spotting those core complaints involves looking at recurring patterns in your own life, then connecting them to possible family history. By differentiating surface-level stuff from core issues and journaling about it, you start to unravel the complex tapestry of your inherited wounds. Give it a shot and watch as your complaints start making more **sense**.

Identifying Core Descriptors

Ever thought about the words you use to talk about yourself and your life? They're more **important** than you might think. The **language** you use says a lot about how you see the world and yourself. This is where identifying core descriptors comes in. It's about spotting those key words and phrases that pop up when you're chatting about your feelings, your past, or even your day-to-day activities.

When you think about it, some words have a way of sticking around. Maybe you call yourself "lazy" when you're feeling down or "lost" when you're unsure about decisions. Pay attention the next time you speak. Are there certain words that always seem to make it into your conversations? Those are your core descriptors. They might seem harmless, but they paint a bigger picture of your inner world. When you identify these words, you start to reveal **patterns** that have been embedded deep inside you, potentially from experiences you've inherited but aren't aware of.

Speaking of patterns, here's a cool idea: "linguistic fingerprints." Basically, these are the unique set of phrases and words we each use that can give away inherited **trauma**. It's like each family hands down a set of emotional narratives along with the family china. Listening to these linguistic fingerprints can be eye-opening. For example, let's say you often say things like "I always mess things up" or "Nothing ever goes my way." These statements can hint at emotional baggage that goes beyond your own lifetime — things possibly transmitted through family history.

Understanding this concept gives you a new way to look at those repeated words, turning them from just annoying habits into clues about deeper issues. Take your time to think about your own phrases. Are there patterns linked to what your parents or even grandparents have said? Maybe your mom often called herself "no good" and now, without realizing, you do the same. It's not so much about the exact words but the emotional beats behind them. Recognizing these can help you begin **healing** from familial patterns.

Here's a fun and practical exercise you can try: the "Word Cloud." Grab a pen and some paper. Write down all the descriptors you use most often to talk about yourself and how you feel. Be honest. Words like "stuck," "happy," "angry," and "confused" all count. Once you've got a good list, head online and use a word cloud generator. You plug in your list, and it will create a visual map of your most frequently used terms. Bigger words mean you use them more often.

Seeing your words in a visual format can have quite an impact. It can highlight what's occupying a lot of space in your mind. If "tired" and "overwhelmed" look much larger in your word cloud, that's a great place to start focusing your healing work. Remember, spotting these core descriptors doesn't mean you have to solve everything right away. It's a way to see clearer and start letting go of what holds you back, step by step.

So, think about these core descriptors. Right? Sit with them. Speak or write them out. Look for the **fingerprints**. Make your word cloud. It's a journey towards freeing yourself from inherited wounds. And trust the **process**. This stuff matters... You matter. And each word you unlock is a step towards a more positive future, without the weight of the past dragging you down.

Discovering Your Core Sentence

You're ready to **figure out** your core sentence. This is the short statement that sums up your deepest fear or belief. Think of it like your emotional shortcut—a quick way to get to the heart of what's weighing you down. We all have those nagging thoughts that keep us up at night. Let's get to the bottom of yours.

Start by thinking about the fears or limiting beliefs that have been hanging around for years. Maybe it's the feeling that you're not good enough. Or that you'll always be abandoned. Everyone's got their own personal ghosts chasing them. What's yours? Close your eyes and let your mind wander over tough moments. Listen to that voice in your head. What does it say over and over?

Try to create a sentence that **captures** that fear or belief in the simplest way you can. Don't overthink it. Just spill it out. Maybe the sentence is "I'm not lovable" or "I'll fail no matter what." These aren't pretty thoughts, but identifying them can set you free.

The reason this core sentence is so important is because it helps you see **patterns** in your family trauma. You may notice that this belief seems to have been passed down from generation to generation. Maybe your parents, grandparents, or even great-grandparents dealt with the same issues. When you notice these connections, it can be a huge relief. You're not just dealing with your issues; you're untangling a web that's been woven over time.

And guess what? Realizing this can **heal** the past while setting the stage for a better future. By confronting these passed-down patterns, you're giving yourself a clean slate.

Next, let's talk about how to really zero in on that belief using the "Sentence Distillation" method. To do this, sit down with a pen and paper, or your phone if that's easier. Jot down the worst things you think about yourself. Don't censor yourself at all.

For instance, you might start with, "I always mess up everything." Then narrow it to, "I'm a mess." Finally, reduce it to something like, "I fail." By boiling it down into one clear sentence, you get a powerful statement that reveals a lot about your internal world at a glance.

This process isn't exactly a walk in the park, be kind to yourself. You might find yourself feeling a bit worn out or emotional. That's okay. That's part of **healing**.

But let's clear something up—it's not just about being aware of this core sentence. It's about what you do after. Once you've whittled your beliefs down to this sentence, start paying attention when it pops up in daily life. Notice how it affects your actions and decisions.

Recognizing this sentence in real time is like flipping a light switch in a dark room. Suddenly, you can see what you're dealing with. And when you know what it is, you can start to **change** it.

So here's to discovering your core sentence. This might seem like a rough bit of work, but it's worth it. Understanding and breaking free from old **trauma** isn't an instant fix, but it's a start. You're laying the groundwork for a future free from inherited emotional baggage. Plain and simple. It's the first step towards building a life where you feel lighter, more free, and heck, maybe even **happy**.

Uncovering Core Traumas

Have you ever noticed how certain words or phrases just seem to **pop up** in your everyday speech? Well, those bits of language can actually help lead you back to specific bad events in your family's past. It's like having your own personal **map** to guide you through the maze of generational trauma. This approach of tracing your main language back to these events is super useful for uncovering stuff that's been lurking around, causing trouble without you even knowing it.

Think about the way you talk, especially when you're **stressed** or upset. Do certain words seem to echo louder than others? These are what we call "trauma echoes." They're like little hints that point to old wounds and unresolved issues from your family history. When someone experiences **trauma**, the way they talk about it or even just the words they use can be passed down, settling into the language of the next generation. Imagine phrases like "I feel trapped" or "Nobody listens to me." They can become part of your main way of talking, hinting at past hurts in your family's story.

So, how do you trace these trauma echoes back to their origins? One handy way is through the "Timeline Tracing" exercise. It's like creating a treasure map, but instead of gold, you're looking for clues to your past. Start by writing down those significant phrases or words you often use. Jotting them down makes them more concrete. From there, you'll want to start **linking** these phrases to different moments in your family's history.

Begin with the easiest way to approach: think about your parents' lives, their stories, stuff you know has happened to them. Did your dad ever complain about feeling stuck at his job, and now you find yourself feeling the same about your career? Write down those stories next to the phrases they might link to. Stories help **bridge** the gap between words and their roots.

Move farther back to your grandparents and beyond, if you can. The stories might get fuzzier or more like myths, but they're still valuable. Maybe there's a tale of your grandma during a rough patch saying something like, "We never had enough," and now you catch yourself worried about financial stability, even when things are going well. Make those connections.

Once you've got this list, you can start to see patterns. It's almost like stepping back and looking at a bigger picture that helps start to understand the sources of your language quirks. What's cool about this process is it's not just dusting off old history – it's making sense of how those old stories still kick around in how we think and talk today.

Given that our language tightly weaves with past traumas, noticing these patterns becomes an eye-opener. But it's also a chance to tweak things. When you catch yourself using those old phrases, dig a bit deeper. Shift them, even slightly. If "trapped" is the echo, adjusting to "I need freedom" starts to open up new **pathways**. You're actively working against the grain of inherited trauma.

In the end, figuring out these core traumas via language and story isn't just a deep-dive into the past. It's also building stepping stones to a brighter future. You're not only honoring where you've come from – you're consciously deciding where to go next.

So, ready to trace your words back to their roots and start shaking off that old **baggage**? Your future self will thank you. Let's start mapping!

Practical Exercise: Creating Your Core Language Map

Let's dive into the good stuff. Creating your Core Language Map starts with **pinpointing** what's bugging you the most in life. What are your most common gripes and complaints? This is crucial because it's like taking out the trash—those recurring annoyances are clues to much deeper things happening within you. So, think about the stuff that keeps popping up in your mind. Is it frustration with always feeling left out? Or maybe you can't stop thinking about how nothing ever goes right for you? Jot these down, even if they seem small or silly.

Think you've listed them all? Great. Now let's move on to the words and phrases you often use. Here's the thing—language has **power**. The way you talk to yourself and describe your life shapes everything. So, what are the words you notice using a lot? Do you catch yourself saying "I can't do this," "This always happens to me," or "What's wrong with me?" again and again? Start making a note of these. You're collecting your core language here, the stuff that's second nature to you but also, sometimes, your own worst enemy.

Now, let's boil all of that down. Pretty daunting, I know. But if you sift through those complaints and words, you'll find a central belief or fear driving them. What's that one sentence that hits right at the heart of it all? Something like "I'm not good enough" or "I'm always alone." This might be hard to admit, but nailing it down is super important. Write it down, so you can really see it.

So, we've figured out your core language, but where does it come from? Let's track it back to your family **history**. Maybe that feeling of "never being good enough" mirrors complaints your parents or grandparents used to voice. Dig into family events or traumas that might have influenced you. Were there life-changing disasters, losses, or patterns of behavior that stood out to you? Start linking your core complaints and words to these past events, and it might start to make sense how some of your own feelings originated.

We're almost there, promise. Let's get visual—time to make a **map**. Grab a piece of paper and put your #1 complaint smack in the middle. Around it, write those common phrases or words you use. Nearby, include that one core sentence you came up with. Finally, draw lines connecting these to the respective family traumas and events you've identified. Soon, you'll see how everything ties together in ways you maybe haven't considered before.

Seeing your Core Language Map laid out might be a **light bulb** moment. Maybe it'll help you understand why you're carrying certain hurts. Don't get discouraged if it feels a bit overwhelming— this map is a powerful tool to start changing those patterns. Next step? Using what you find to start the real **healing** work.

In Conclusion

This chapter has shown how **vital** it is to understand and articulate the deep-seated **beliefs** and **traumas** inherited from your family. By recognizing the **language** you use—your core complaints, descriptors, and sentences—you can trace these patterns back to their origins and begin to **transform** your experiences. Remember, the words you speak are powerful reflections of your inner world.

You've seen the importance of identifying your most recurring life **complaints** and their deep family roots. Surface-level grievances often mask deeper issues, and there's real benefit in recognizing key words and phrases you use to describe yourself. You've learned how to create a concise statement that embodies your main fear or belief, and you've explored the **connection** between core language and family history through specific events.

Understanding these concepts gives you the power to see and change the **narratives** that have long influenced you. Apply these insights daily, and you'll start noticing patterns that reveal deeper truths about yourself and your family history. This awareness is the first step towards a brighter, more self-aware future. Keep exploring and addressing these core language patterns to make meaningful changes in your life.

Chapter 6: Releasing Emotional Baggage

Ever wonder what life would be like without the **weight** of the past holding you down? In this chapter, I've laid out a **toolkit** just for you, aiming to clear the emotional fog you've carried for years. Trust me, I've been there—dragging old pains around, not realizing how they shaped my today.

Imagine a new you, free from inherited **pain** and generational **guilt**. It's about time you let go, right? Together, we'll explore fresh emotional patterns and practical steps to shed all the **turmoil** that's been bogging you down. Yeah, it might sound a bit daunting, but aren't you curious about the **peace** this change might bring? Picture more relaxed days, feeling lighter, more at ease.

And don't worry—I've included an easy **exercise** to help ground these changes in real life. With each step, you'll feel the shift, a tangible **lightness**. Ready? Let's dive in.

Acknowledging Inherited Pain

You know that old saying, "The apple doesn't fall far from the tree"? Well, it's true for our **emotions** too. Start by noticing the emotional patterns within your family. Do you often feel sadness even when everything seems fine? Or maybe there's a constant worry that lingers without any specific cause. These feelings might not be your own. They could be the emotional baggage you're carrying from past generations.

Take a look at your family's **history**. Think about the stories told by your parents, grandparents, and even great-grandparents. Were there experiences of war, loss, or hardship? Those experiences can leave emotional scars. Just like physical traits, these can be passed down through generations. It's called "ancestral grief" – the idea that emotional pain isn't just yours but shared in your lineage.

Imagine your ancestors' pain stored in an emotional bank. Over time, those unresolved feelings get passed down. This concept explains why you might feel certain emotions intensely without a clear personal reason. By understanding this, you can validate those feelings and start working through them.

An essential tool in this acknowledgment process is the "Emotional Inheritance **Inventory**." It's like a checklist where you map out the emotional patterns inherited from your family. Start by writing down recurring emotions you feel – sadness, anxiety, anger, or fear. Next, jot down the stories of family members who might have experienced similar feelings. Soon, you'll start seeing patterns.

Here's what you can do:

• Identify basic emotions you frequently have without specific triggers.

• Reflect on common emotional themes in family stories.

• Map out where these emotions might intersect in your family history.

This inventory becomes a powerful acknowledgment tool since seeing it in writing validates your feelings. You realize these emotions aren't inexplicable burdens but inherited and open to understanding.

Think of a smooth lake - still on the surface but deep underneath. Your emotions might seem unmanageable, but acknowledging them helps you explore these depths with purpose. Now that you see how this inherited pain influences you, it opens the door to start addressing it. Shifting from blaming yourself toward understanding reduces unnecessary **guilt**. This small shift changes how you tackle these deep-rooted feelings.

When you see this bigger picture, **relationships** make more sense. You might get why certain topics trigger your parents or siblings. Think about those moments where the family dynamic suddenly shifts – often, it's those inherited patterns acting out. Validating this not only soothes personal pain but fosters better understanding and connection with loved ones.

Picking up the pieces of your family's emotional past is not always easy, but it's crucial for **healing**. Picture stepping into a dimly lit room... you flick on the light, revealing cluttered boxes and memories – that's what acknowledging inherited pain does. By illuminating this room, you begin to see both the clutter and space available to create something new.

Moving forward, approach your Emotional Inheritance Inventory frequently. This isn't something done once – your emotional landscape shifts as you grow and learn. Keep noting new emotions or revisiting old patterns. Doing this makes these feelings less powerful. You're no longer taken by surprise because you've mapped out why they exist.

Simply unearthing where these emotions come from helps clear the path towards healing. Understanding ancestral grief helps demystify and validate present feelings. With your Emotional Inheritance Inventory, you gain **clarity** and start taking those first steps away from inherited pain towards building a positive, self-defined emotional **future**.

Letting Go of Generational Guilt

Taking on family **guilt** can feel like carrying someone else's weight in your backpack. It's heavy, frustrating, and, to be honest, a bit nonsense since it isn't your baggage to begin with. So, let's find ways to let go of that guilt tied to family **trauma** and those patterns passed down through generations.

Sometimes you might think, wrongly so, that the struggles and missteps of your parents or grandparents are your fault. This mindset traps you in a state of feeling responsible for things beyond your control. Why should you take the hit for choices you didn't make? Inherited patterns and traumas often confuse you, making you think you're to blame for years of hardship. It's like taking the blame for a leaking roof just because you're living in the house now. Understanding this can help you step back and see things clearly.

Alright, so let's break up this idea of "misplaced **responsibility**" around generational trauma. It's like a weird game of tag where you never agreed to play, but somehow you're it. You might look back at family issues and think, "If I had just been different," or, "Maybe if I had done that." But that responsibility isn't yours. It's the difference between being a player and being a spectator at the game - you're on a different team. You wouldn't expect spectators to score goals or make plays. So, why accept blame for actions not in your control?

Now, switch your focus to letting this misguided guilt go. Right, let's work through a "Guilt Release" **visualization** technique. It may sound a bit woo-woo, but stay with me here—sometimes a symbolic gesture can make a big difference. Close your eyes and picture a suitcase. This suitcase holds all that inherited guilt, packed away by your ancestors. Now imagine yourself opening this suitcase. See the items inside, representing different guilt aspects: a rusted key, old letters, maybe even heavy stones. With each breath out, remove one item and set it on the ground next to you, letting that weight slip away. The suitcase now gets lighter. When empty, close it, lock it, and toss the key. Watch the suitcase dissolve or blow away like dust on the wind. And feel the guilt blowing away, too.

This method may not wipe away guilt in one go. It requires practice and patience. See this as part of a habit of mind-clearing and emotionally cleansing. When those guilty thoughts creep back, repeat the visualization—even in quick ten-second bursts. Over time, allow those harsh, deeply ingrained **emotions** to loosen their hold on you.

Taking the process steady, you'll find more **empathy** towards yourself and a clearer mind. It's a bit like giving yourself breathing room after being wrapped too tight in invisible strings. Only when you shed this unwelcome weight can you start living genuinely and freely, without constantly checking over your shoulder for guilt that doesn't belong to you.

So, don't rush, but know it's okay to let go of things that don't help you. Holding onto **pain** and guilt handed down through family lines won't make anyone's past hurt less. But it does make your present and **future** lighter and brighter. Now, doesn't that sound more inviting?

Forgiving Yourself and Your Ancestors

Healing from family **trauma** isn't just about looking forward. It's also about looking back with a sense of softness and kindness toward yourself—and your ancestors. When you develop **compassion** for yourself and the folks who came before, you open up a path to true healing. You start to see the pain that passed down through the generations and understand that everyone did the best they could with what they had.

Developing self-compassion isn't easy, though. You might think back on your own struggles and feel anger, guilt, or shame. But take a moment and **breathe**. Instead of beating yourself up for feeling this way, try to recognize the part of you that wants to protect yourself. This part means well but doesn't always know how to let go of the pain. And that's where compassion steps in. Imagine talking to yourself like you would to a close buddy who's having a rough time. Remind yourself that it's okay to feel hurt. It's okay to have complicated emotions.

When thinking about your ancestors and their struggles, try to remember that they, too, were doing their best. Life many years ago wasn't any easier—and often it was much harder. Picture them facing their own problems, sometimes making choices that weren't so great because they didn't know any better. Showing them this kind of understanding creates a sense of connection and humanity. It recognizes their flaws and their hurt while opening the door to let go of what no longer serves you.

Feeling compassion naturally leads you to **forgiveness**. It's like a bridge that connects your current self to your past and future. Forgiveness is a powerful tool for breaking cycles of generational trauma. By forgiving those who came before you, you release the grip that old pain can still have on you. It doesn't mean forgetting or saying that the past wasn't hurtful. Instead, it's about freeing your heart from carrying burdens that aren't yours to bear anymore.

Forgiveness reshapes how you see your own **story**. It reframes the narrative from one of an endless loop of hurt to one where healing and growth are possible. When you forgive your ancestors, you stop the cycle of guilt and misery and create new ways of being for yourself and those who come after you. You become the change-maker in your family's story.

Which brings us to a powerful exercise—writing an "Ancestral Forgiveness" **letter**. This might sound a bit different, but it's a fantastic way to express your understanding and start letting go of what's been weighing you down. Grab a pen and paper, and sit somewhere quiet. Imagine you're writing to one of your ancestors, maybe someone whose life choices have directly impacted you.

In your letter, write about how their struggles and choices affected you and how you feel about it. Allow yourself to be honest and open with your feelings. Next, consider what they might have been facing in their time. Write down any thoughts of understanding or sympathy that come to mind. Lastly, express your forgiveness. Tell them you're ready to let go of the hurt and anger. Here's an example to get you started:

"Dear [Ancestor's Name],

I've been thinking a lot about how your life has shaped mine. I know you had your battles, and I've felt the sting of choices you made. But I've come to understand that you were grappling with your pain and challenges. It must have been so hard for you. I want to let you know that I **forgive** you. I'm choosing to release this pain from my heart. Thank you for the lessons, and I hope you find peace just as I'm finding mine."

Use this template to guide your thoughts. Writing it all out can be incredibly freeing. It helps you articulate thoughts and emotions you might not have known were lingering inside. With this step taken, you pave the way to a lighter, more positive future for yourself and the generations ahead.

Creating New Emotional Patterns

Alright, so you're ready to take **control** of your emotions—a really brave step. You're going to learn how to consciously choose and grow new emotional responses. It's like starting a new garden. You remove the old weeds, prepare the soil, and plant seeds that will grow into beautiful flowers. In this case, those old weeds are the unwanted emotional responses you inherited, and the seeds are the new, positive ones you'll learn to nurture.

Let's start by acknowledging that it's perfectly normal to repeat emotional patterns you've seen in your family. It's sort of automatic because you've been seeing them for so long. But guess what? You have the **power** to change this. Begin by identifying specific reactions you want to change. For instance, if you always feel overly anxious during family gatherings because that's how you saw your parents react, pinpoint that anxiety. This moment of recognition is the starting point.

So what now? Imagine you're crafting a completely new response. You might think of yourself as an artist, painting on a blank canvas. Start by practicing small changes. If you feel that twinge of anxiety creeping up, pause, take a breath, and consciously pick a calmer emotion. It won't be perfect the first time, and that's okay. This is all about **practice**.

And let's talk about "emotional reprogramming"—a fancy term, but really, it's not complicated. Think of your brain as a computer with software installed by your past experiences. Some of these programs are helpful, like kindness and love. Others, not so much. Emotional reprogramming is about updating that software.

Similar to when you update an app on your phone, you recognize a pattern isn't working well, go through the process to change it, and install a better version. Simple, right? Start by observing your **thoughts**. Every time an old, unhelpful thought pops up, gently push it aside and introduce a new, positive one. It's a back-and-forth game between the old and the new. Gradually, the new thoughts will grow stronger, much like muscles getting stronger with exercise.

Now, moving on to something super practical—the "Pattern Interruption" technique. This is handy for breaking usual emotional reactions that don't serve you well. Think of it as hitting the pause button when you start feeling an old, unwanted emotion. When you're about to fall into an old pattern, do something unexpected. Clap your hands, hum a tune, or even take a silly dance break. This interruption creates a momentary break in your habitual response, giving you the space to choose a different **emotion**.

Imagine you're at a family dinner, and Aunt Sally makes her usual critical comment. You feel anger or hurt rising. Instead of reacting, interrupt it—clap your hands lightly, hum for a second, or take three deep breaths. This small act disrupts the cycle, letting you pick a different reaction, maybe humor or indifference.

While Pattern Interruption is great in the moment, combining it with emotional reprogramming makes it even more powerful. Each time you interrupt a pattern and choose a better reaction, you're also reprogramming your brain to default to the newer, healthier **response**.

It's a bit like training a puppy—consistent and gentle corrections do wonders. Just as you'd reward your pup for good behavior, give yourself mental pats on the back when you adopt a new emotional response.

So, the **journey** to emotional freedom isn't a straight path. It's full of twists, turns, and probably a few setbacks. But each conscious choice puts you closer to a more positive, emotionally fulfilling life. And let's face it, that's worth every **effort**, isn't it?

Here's the revised and refined text:

Practical Exercise: Emotional Release Ritual

Ready to **unleash** your pent-up emotions? This simple yet **powerful** ritual might be just what you need. Grab a pen and paper, find a quiet spot, and let's get started.

First, take a few deep **breaths** to center yourself. Now, think about a situation that's been bothering you lately. It could be anything from a minor annoyance to a major life event. As you reflect, allow yourself to really **feel** those emotions.

Start **writing** down everything that comes to mind. Don't hold back – this is your chance to let it all out. Curse, rant, or even draw angry faces if that helps. The goal is to **express** yourself fully and honestly.

Once you've gotten it all out on paper, take a moment to **acknowledge** your feelings. They're valid, and it's okay to have them. Now comes the **cathartic** part: carefully tear up the paper into tiny pieces. As you do this, imagine you're releasing those negative emotions.

Finally, dispose of the torn paper. You can throw it away, flush it down the toilet, or even burn it safely if you're feeling dramatic. The physical act of destroying the paper symbolizes letting go of those emotions.

Remember, this exercise isn't about suppressing your feelings. It's about processing them in a healthy way and then moving forward. You might find it helpful to do this regularly, especially when you're feeling overwhelmed or stuck.

Give it a try and see how it works for you. You might be surprised at how much lighter you feel afterward.

In Conclusion

In this chapter, you've learned some **essential** ways to let go of inherited emotional baggage and lighten your emotional load. This process involves recognizing the emotional pains handed down through generations and finding the inner **strength** to release them.

It's about understanding where your feelings come from and transforming them for a healthier, happier future.

You've seen how to recognize inherited emotions and their origins, and you've gained insight into **understanding ancestral grief** and how it affects your current feelings. You've learned to create an "Emotional Inheritance Inventory" to track emotional patterns, discovered **strategies** to release guilt tied to family trauma, and practiced forgiveness for yourself and your ancestors to break emotional cycles.

By applying what you've learned, you can start a **healing** process that allows you to grow and create new, positive emotional patterns. Take the time to reflect on what emotions you carry and choose to let go. You have the **power** to transform your emotional world into one filled with more joy and peace.

Remember, this journey is unique to you. As you work through your inherited emotions, be patient with yourself. It's okay to take small steps and celebrate each **milestone** along the way. Your emotional well-being is worth the effort, and the **rewards** of this work can be life-changing.

Now, go ahead and put these techniques into practice for a brighter future! You've got this, mate!

Chapter 7: Healing the Inner Child

Ever **wondered** why certain things from your past still sting? It's about time you look at **healing** those old wounds. You ever feel like the **child** you once were is still hanging around, needing some love? This chapter is all about **reconnecting** with that younger self and giving it the care it deserves. You're gonna take a journey—with me showing the way and you doing the brave **work**—to make things right.

Can you imagine having a **chat** with yourself as a kid, giving comforting insights? Trust me, the **rewards** of reparenting and self-nurturing are worth every moment. Plus, once you've learned these techniques, think about how much stronger and more **resilient** your inner child will become. With some practical exercises included, you're not just reading—you're actually doing something about it. Let's get started on this meaningful path together.

Reconnecting with Your Younger Self

Ever **thought** about your younger self, the one who loved cartoons and had big dreams? Connecting with those stages of your childhood can help deal with family **trauma**. The child in you forgets easily, but that doesn't mean the memories and feelings are gone.

Looking at old **photos** is a good start. Pictures tell a lot. That little you had fears, joys, and felt things deeply. Try to remember how each photo makes you feel. Was there a time when you felt really safe and loved? Or moments when you felt misunderstood? Those memories matter. Talk to yourself in those photos. Sometimes your younger self might answer back with thoughts and feelings.

Think about different ages. Five-year-old you may need different healing than teen you. **Childhood** comes in stages. Each stage might have different wounds or happy moments. It's like reading a book with different chapters, each having its own story. Was there a happy eight-year-old you? Or a sad twelve-year-old feeling alone? Knowing these different stages helps spot where healing is needed.

Shine a light on those hidden moments. Life events that seemed small back then could've had a huge impact. Remembering these can be key to **healing**.

But why does this matter? This whole "inner child work" might seem kinda weird, right? Actually, it's vital for fixing those old family wounds that stick around in adult life. Often, problems you face trace back to things that happened years ago. When you're angry at your dad for something small, maybe it's really about something that happened when you were ten. Or maybe, there's an old wound from your mom that you're projecting on present relationships. Reconnecting helps face these hidden pains staring you in your adulthood.

Simply put, what happened back then affects what you do now. Ever snap at someone and wonder why? Digging into these old wounds reveals habits and **reactions** formed years ago. By healing these, you can change your present reactions. Because if you don't tackle these head-on, they fuel responses and decisions all your life. And let's be real, nobody wants their five-year-old self running their life.

Alright, you're convinced but wondering how to kick off this inner child work. Ever tried Age Regression techniques? They're great for diving back into childhood. Find a quiet spot. Close your eyes and picture a safe place - a garden, a cozy room, wherever you felt happy once. Focus. Now, imagine a younger you appearing there. What do they look like? How do they feel? Start talking to them. Ask about their day, worries, what makes them laugh.

You might say, "Hi little buddy, what's bothering you?" Or, "Hey man, why are you sad today?" The goal is to get them to talk. Let them lead the **conversation**. Keep it casual. You're an older brother here, ready to listen. Watch the feelings emerge, good or bad. If a bad memory pops up, don't freak out. Stay calm. Offer reassurance to this younger self. Remind them they're safe with you.

So there it is, connecting with your younger self and why it matters. Start with old pictures, remember the stages, dive into those hidden **memories**. Getting through this, addressing the past instead of running from it? That's how the healing begins for present you and future you. After all, kid you deserves that relief.

Addressing Childhood Wounds

Healing childhood wounds is like unraveling an old, knotted ball of yarn. It takes time to notice each thread - something that was perhaps overlooked for years. You might not even realize how many **wounds** are there. Recognizing specific childhood **traumas** is the first step. Think back to times you felt ignored or dismissed, or times you felt scared without comfort. Maybe there were moments no one celebrated you or when you felt stifled and couldn't speak up. All these experiences sit quietly but shape who you are today.

Little by little, these wounds affect your **behavior**. For instance, if you were often ignored, you might find yourself overachieving now to gain approval. Think about this: ever felt anxious when someone's mad at you? That could be a sign of past experiences resurfacing. These old wounds also creep into **relationships**.

Imagine expecting your partner to figure out you're upset without you saying a word. When they don't, it stings twice as much. Sometimes, childhood wounds make you depend too much on others or, the opposite, make you build walls too high for anyone to climb.

Let's do an activity to pinpoint these hurt spots, called "Wound Mapping." Find a quiet space and a piece of paper. Draw a person in the middle—that's you. Now, around this figure, write down moments you think might be wounds. They don't have to be terrible incidents. Small things matter too. Maybe your parents argued on Christmas, and you hate holidays because of it. Whatever pops in your head is worth writing down. Take your time and jot every thought that seems relevant, fill up the sheet if you need.

Next, let's connect these moments to current behaviors and feelings. Draw lines from each childhood wound to how they manifest in your present life. Say, if you wrote about feeling unnoticed as a child, you might draw a line to current feelings of insignificance at work. Once you spot these patterns, it's easier to untangle them. Every line is like a connection to a present-day struggle born from a past hurt.

Don't rush this process; map as much as you need. **Healing** isn't a sprint. It's a gentle walk through your personal history. Keep in mind that doing this may bring up emotions. Allow yourself to feel whatever comes up. You deserve that compassion. These feelings are pointers to where the knots are that need careful loosening. This isn't about blaming anybody—it's about understanding where the wounds come from.

These wounds, once acknowledged, start the journey of healing. Like they say, knowing is half the battle. Post-wound mapping, reflect on these connections often. It might surprise you how patterns from your past keep showing up in ways you didn't realize. The road to healing begins with this realization, slowly guiding you towards a life less burdened by the past and more open to a brighter tomorrow.

So, next time, if you notice a **behavior** that doesn't align with who you want to be, consider its origins. Do you see a connection to a mapped wound? Recognizing that link could be the key to changing it. It's not just about patching hurts. It's about growing through and beyond them, creating a new **narrative**, a lighter one, with each recognition and each healed moment. You're doing the work. You're healing the child that once was, shaping a better future self with understanding and care. Keep at it; every bit counts.

Reparenting Techniques for Self-Nurturing

Developing a **caring** inner voice is key to counteracting bad childhood messages. It might feel strange at first, I know it did for me. Those old messages, the ones that whisper you're not good enough or you're unlovable, can be loud. But guess what? You can teach yourself a new way to talk to yourself. It's like being your own **cheerleader** instead of your harsher critic.

Start with simple, kind words. Think about what you'd say to a close friend struggling. "You're doing the best you can," or "It's okay to make mistakes." Try saying these things to yourself, even if it feels awkward. Over time, this new voice starts to feel more natural. It's like cleaning up a messy room—a little effort each day, and eventually, you have a more comfortable space.

Now, let's dive into the idea of "**self-parenting**." This isn't just talking nice to yourself. It's about taking on the role of the parent you might have needed when you were younger. That means setting healthy boundaries, making sure you get enough rest, or giving yourself permission to enjoy life without guilt. In many ways, you become your own caretaker.

Visualizing yourself as both the child and the parent can be powerful. Think about what younger you would need. Maybe it's a hug, reassurance, or even just the permission to play. Now, give those gifts to yourself. This might look like taking a break when you're tired or seeking out a friend when you need support. Gradually, you'll notice a shift in how you **care** for yourself, nurturing your younger self's needs.

Okay, here's where it gets more practical. The "Inner Dialogue" technique is a **game-changer** for practicing positive self-talk. Start by writing down those negative messages you hear in your head. Got them? Now, respond to them as the caring parent. If your inner critic says, "You'll never succeed," respond with, "It's okay to feel scared, but I believe in you. We can take small steps towards our goal."

It's almost like having a conversation with yourself. At first, it may seem a bit odd, but I promise—it works. It teaches you to provide your own **emotional** support, turning harsh criticisms into opportunities for encouragement. As you practice this, you'll start to notice a subtle but powerful shift. The negative comments lose their sting because you've learned to counter them with compassion.

Developing these habits won't happen overnight. It's a process of daily small steps—replacing one bad thought at a time with a nurturing one. Imagine you've been plucking out the weeds and planting flowers instead. Over time, a beautiful **garden** grows.

Learning to nurture yourself through a caring inner voice, self-parenting, and positive self-talk is all about practice and patience. You're not reshaping inherited wounds alone; you're also creating a healthier, happier future for yourself. Keep at it, and bit by bit, you'll find the old, harmful messages fading into the background, replaced by the voice of someone who genuinely **cares** for you: you.

Building Inner Child Resilience

A **strong** inner child doesn't just appear out of thin air. It takes some effort, but you can definitely make it happen. You just need to build up that emotional toughness. Think of it like teaching a kid to ride a bike. You can start by focusing on boosting your inner child's **resilience**.

To get the ball rolling, it's crucial to create moments where your inner child feels supported and safe. Imagine having a heart-to-heart with that younger version of yourself. What would they need to hear to feel stronger? Maybe it's words of encouragement, like "You're **capable**," or "You're loved no matter what." Positive affirmations create a foundation of trust and love where your inner child can flourish.

Another way is by remembering past tough times that you managed to get through. Reflect on these experiences, and remind your inner self that they can overcome anything. These reflections **strengthen** your inner child, showing them that even when faced with challenges, they can bounce back.

What if your inner child didn't get the nurturing they needed when you were young? This is where "retroactive nurturing" comes in. It lets you go back and give yourself that care you missed out on. Picture a **memory** where you felt alone or scared. Step into that memory, but this time, bring your present-day self into it. Be there as your own guardian angel. Imagine hugging your younger self, offering comforting words, and promising protection.

In these moments, visualize filling the gap of that emotional neglect. Maybe sit with your inner child in a safe place, like a favorite childhood spot. Keep talking to them softly, assuring safety and love. Doing this helps repair old wounds, making strides to fix the neglect once and for all. This reclaiming of old hurts can allow **healing** to seep into the past, affecting your entire timeline.

Now, let's dive into the "Resilience Building" **visualization**. This exercise works wonders. Start by finding a comfy, quiet place where you can sit undisturbed. Close your eyes and take a few deep breaths. Imagine a place where you always feel safe. This could be a real place you've been to or something entirely from your imagination. Get settled in this place.

Now, bring in your inner child. Visualize them feeling happy and secure in this environment. Create some positive activities around them - maybe they're playing, laughing, or exploring safely. Introduce supportive figures into the scene like imaginary friends, gentle animals, or wise guardians. Make sure this place is filled with warmth, colors, and sounds that are comforting.

As the scene builds up, envision a glowing shield around them. This represents that untouchable resilience. The more detailed you make this visualization, the stronger this protective aura gets. Let your inner child know that this safe haven is always available for them, and they can always retreat here for comfort and **strength** throughout life's trials.

Combining these strategies will nurture resilience within your inner child. Creating a positive inner atmosphere, healing past wounds with retroactive nurturing, and practicing the resilience-building visualization set strong foundations. It's like forming a well-rounded team of supportive guides in your head. When your inner child feels seen and valued, the emotional toughness flourishes naturally over time. Don't rush it—take it one step at a time, and keep nourishing that inner world with love and compassion.

Practical Exercise: Inner Child Dialogue

Finding a quiet, comfy spot and closing your eyes sounds simple, right? It's your start to **healing**. Settle in somewhere you won't be disturbed. You're about to go on a meaningful journey. Close your eyes and take a breath. Feel the air entering your lungs, then slowly leaving...like a gentle wave. This space is yours—safe and calm.

Now, picture your **inner child**. Is this tiny you from your childhood? Or maybe an older version during a rough phase? How old are you in this image? Picture as much detail as you can—clothing, surroundings, even emotions you felt back then. You might feel a lump in your throat. It's okay, sit with it. This is where the magic begins.

Starting a mental chat with your inner child may feel odd at first, but it's a way to connect with past hurts and needs. Ask questions. What does this young version of you need? Ask gently, maybe starting with, "Hey, what's bothering you?" or "What can I do to help?" Listen without judgement. Your inner child might need love, understanding, or even a reminder of safety.

Listening and replying with kindness is crucial. Hear what this younger you is saying. Maybe share comforting words like, "I'm here for you" or "I understand you." It's like talking to a beloved little one. Respond with patience. These words healing old wounds become bridges between what was and what can be.

Giving comfort, support, and reassurance moves to soothing old hurts. Tell your inner child that they're loved and valued. Simple phrases like, "You're safe" or "You're strong" can be massively comforting. Hold on to these moments; making your past self feel valued heals old wounds and nurtures new **strength**.

Now, picture **hugging** your inner child. This act symbolizes merging your past and present selves. Imagine your arms holding that younger version. Feeling the connection bridging time might stir feelings, but also deep comfort. Envision the blend of hurts and strengths...past melting into you now.

Opening your eyes, jot down insights and feelings from this experience. What did your inner child say? How did you respond?

Write down anything you felt—thoughts, memories, even small words or phrases. This captures raw **emotions**, sealing in the progress you've made.

By following each step thoughtfully, you'll foster an intimate **dialogue** with your inner child, promoting healing and growth. This exercise isn't about achieving perfection in one sitting...it'll be messy, touching knots in your heart. But with each practice, you'll knit together the frayed threads of your past, creating a wrap of understanding and compassion for yourself.

Picturing this inner dialogue as a regular practice will contribute to deeper healing, bit by bit. Embracing this step-by-step process opens **communication** channels within yourself...one healing conversation at a time. Keep these interactions alive and listen to your responses with patience and love...each time strengthening this vital relationship with your inner child.

In Conclusion

In this chapter, we've **explored** the ways to heal and reconnect with your inner child. Remember, understanding and nurturing past hurt can lead to a healthier, happier you. From understanding different stages of your childhood, addressing hidden **wounds**, to practicing tender self-care—each step moves you closer to emotional well-being.

You've seen the **importance** of connecting with different stages of your childhood and learned what "inner child work" means and why it matters. We've covered how to use the "Age Regression" technique to visit childhood **memories**, and discussed strategies to recognize and heal childhood traumas. You've also gained insight into how childhood pain affects adult **behavior** and relationships.

Taking these lessons to heart can truly **transform** how you feel about yourself. Practice the techniques we've learned and start nurturing the most significant person in your life—yourself. You have the **power** to heal and create a brighter future!

Remember, this journey is uniquely yours. As you continue to work on yourself, be patient and kind. Your inner child has been waiting for your attention, and now you're equipped to give it the care it deserves. Embrace this process, and watch as your **relationships** improve and your self-understanding deepens. You've got this!

Chapter 8: Transforming Family Relationships

Ever wonder why **family** can both lift you up and drag you down? I've been there too. In this chapter, you'll discover ways to make real **changes** in how you deal with your relatives. Think of it as a roadmap to peace around the dinner table.

I'll guide you through setting **boundaries** so your relationships stay healthy. You'll get to work on improving how you and your family **communicate** with each other. Ever had a family argument that never really got settled? We'll tackle those nagging **issues** too. Plus, you'll pick up tips for giving and receiving emotional **support** from those closest to you.

So if you're ready to fix what's broken and build something better, keep reading. This chapter is all about **transformation**, and you're gonna love how it feels to get closer to the ones you care about. Ready to dive in?

You'll learn how to:

• Establish clear boundaries without causing friction

• Enhance your communication skills for better family dynamics

• Address long-standing conflicts and find resolutions

• Cultivate a supportive environment within your family

By the end of this chapter, you'll have the tools to create more **meaningful** connections with your loved ones. So, buckle up and get ready for a journey that'll transform your family relationships for the better!

Setting Healthy Boundaries with Family

Setting **boundaries** with family isn't always a walk in the park. It's tough when you want to keep the peace, but you also need to look out for yourself. Here's how to spot and stick to your own boundaries in family situations.

First, figure out what your limits are. Pay attention to how you feel when you're around family. Do you feel **overwhelmed** or stressed out? Those feelings can be clues that your boundaries are being crossed. For example, if you feel anxious when your cousin brings up certain topics, that's a sign. Or if your mom's constant calling bugs you, that's another clue. Defining these boundaries isn't about shutting people out—it's about protecting your well-being.

Once you've spotted the signs, it's time to take **action**. You've got to communicate your boundaries clearly and respectfully. If your brother tends to call late at night and it disrupts your sleep, let him know daytime calls are better. It's all about talking it out before things get fuzzy and line-blurry. Be firm but kind; you're not aiming to start a feud, just to create space for yourself.

Next, stick to your guns. It's not enough to set the boundaries; you've got to **enforce** them. If your mom calls at 11 PM and you've already had the "no late calls" talk, don't answer the phone. It might feel harsh at first, but it's necessary. You might slip up sometimes, letting things slide, and that's okay. The important thing is to keep trying and remain consistent.

But you know what can make all this a bit trickier? **Emotional enmeshment**. This one's a doozy and can majorly affect family ties.

Emotional enmeshment happens when family members blur the lines between their own emotions and identities with each other's. It's like everyone has their fingers in everybody else's emotional business, making it super tough to figure out where you end and another begins. If your sister always feels your problems as if they were hers, or you find yourself stressed out because your dad is, you might be emotionally enmeshed. It's draining and makes setting boundaries look like rocket science.

To tackle emotional enmeshment, you'll need to develop a stronger sense of **self**. Get to know who you really are, outside the family dynamic. Take up solo activities that you enjoy without the family influence. Simple acts like going for a walk or reading in solitude can help. Sometimes, you might even need to explain to family members what enmeshment is. It can feel like a can of worms, but it's necessary.

Transitioning from understanding emotional enmeshment brings us right to the crucial step—actually setting these boundaries with a script.

You might find it useful to have a "Boundary Setting" **script** when you talk to your family about what you need. This can make the conversation easier and less prone to going off-track.

Here's a script you could use:

"I really appreciate how much you care about me, and that's why this conversation is so important. I've noticed I feel overwhelmed when __ (insert specific situation). I need to have __ (insert boundary), so I can feel better and be my best self around you all. I hope you can understand and support this."

Fill in the blanks with your specific issues and boundaries. Don't miss the appreciation part—it makes the request less like a demand and more about mutual respect. Stick to the script or adapt where necessary, just ensure it's clear.

There you have it—by spotting boundary issues, understanding emotional enmeshment, and using a clear script, you can transform family **interactions** and create healthier relationships. It'll take practice and patience. But even small steps lead to big changes over time.

Improving Communication Patterns

Talking to family can feel like running in circles sometimes, right? Well, **spotting** bad communication habits is the first step to fixing them. Have you ever noticed how a simple misunderstanding spirals into a full-blown argument? That's because of these habits. Things like interrupting, not really listening, and always needing to be right can muck up even the best intentions.

So how do you spot these habits? Pay attention. When someone is talking, resist the urge to jump in with your point. Instead, just **listen**. Notice if you're thinking about your response while they're still speaking. If you are, you're probably not fully engaged. This is a sign of bad communication.

Then there's the issue of always needing to get the last word in. This habit often makes the conversation more about winning than about understanding. Try to let go of that need. You'll find that more harmonious chats follow.

Moving on, let's talk about something called "**circular** communication." Imagine two people arguing and consistently falling into the same patterns. One person throws out an old grievance, the other responds defensively, and around and around they go. It's like being stuck on a carousel that just won't stop.

To break free from this cycle, it's important to recognize when it's happening. Take a step back and **assess** the conversation. Does it feel like you're just rehashing the same points? That means you're in a circular pattern. So, how do you stop it? Change the way you respond. Instead of reacting defensively, acknowledge the grievance. Say something like, "I understand you're upset because..." It's tough at first, but this shift can help steer the conversation onto a productive path.

Now, let's dig into a technique that can help you understand and be understood: **Active** Listening. It's more than just hearing words—it's about really getting what the other person is saying. When you practice active listening, you're fully present.

Here's how to do it. When someone else speaks, focus completely on them. Don't let your mind drift to your own agenda. Make little verbal nods—"I see," "Go on," "That makes sense"—to show you're engaged. Repeat back key points occasionally. For example, say, "So, you're saying that..." to confirm you've understood correctly. This not only shows you're paying attention but also helps clarify any potential misunderstandings on the spot.

Comparing active listening to just hearing, it's evident how much more **positive** the interaction becomes. Folks feel valued when they know you're genuinely focused on them. This builds **empathy**, which naturally smooths over those tricky family dynamics.

Transitioning smoothly, let's connect the idea of breaking circular communication to improving listening skills. Both focus on changing ingrained habits to shift the tone of your interactions towards understanding.

Ultimately, enhancing **communication** with family involves keen observation, stepping back from old patterns, and diving deep into genuinely attentive listening. Try out these tactics and feel the change. It's not about winning arguments; it's about building a new, positive way to relate to each other.

Addressing Unresolved Family Conflicts

Family conflicts are pretty much like those old scars—you really want them gone, but don't always know where to start. Old fights with family can hang around for a long time. But there are ways to handle and fix these long-standing issues. Let's get into it.

So, you've got some family fights that have been going on forever. Ignoring them? Not really solving anything. Here's what you can do:

• **Start** a Conversation: Yup, talk. Sounds simple, right? Well, it's got to be more than just words. You need to have honest, open conversations. Set aside time to really talk about what's been bugging you and others. No interruptions. No blaming.

• Listen Up: Seriously, really listen to what the other person is saying. Put yourself in their shoes, even if their perspective is tough to swallow.

• Keep It Cool: **Emotions** run high in these talks, so keep things calm. If things get heated, take a break and come back. There's no rush.

But how do you understand these conflicts better? That's where Family Systems Theory comes in.

Family Systems Theory isn't just some obscure concept. It's a way to look at family problems by seeing the family as a whole, where each member plays a part. Imagine each person's actions affecting everyone else, like cogs turning in a machine. Fix one part, and the whole machine works smoother.

For example, maybe your sibling's nagging isn't just to annoy you. It might be their way of showing concern. Seeing it from this angle can change how you react. You're not just looking at your side, but how everyone's pieces fit together.

So, now you're thinking about the whole family system and realizing how one person's issue can impact everyone else. This brings us to a handy tool—**Conflict** Mapping.

Conflict Mapping is like making a map of the issues and connections in your family. But instead of roads and rivers, you're charting relationships and conflicts.

Here's how to do it:

• Grab Some Paper: Start by writing everyone's name down on a big piece of paper. Family members, close relatives—anyone involved.

• Draw **Connections**: Draw lines between people who have conflicts or strong bonds. Different colors can show fights or friendships.

• Pinpoint the Issues: Next to each line, jot down what the core issue is. Jealousy? Misunderstanding? Maybe it's something specific like money matters.

• Look for Patterns: Are there patterns? Certain people that seem to have more conflicts? This can help to see if maybe there's a deeper, root cause.

• Brainstorm **Solutions**: Now, for each issue, think of one small step you could take. Maybe it's having another calm conversation. Maybe it's agreeing to disagree on certain topics.

By mapping things out, you get a clearer picture of the whole setup. Things that seemed really tangled can start making sense, and solutions that were hidden might become obvious.

Tackling long-standing family issues is no walk in the park, but it doesn't have to feel impossible either. Start those conversations, understand the whole system, and use conflict mapping to get a grip on the tricky parts of family **relationships**. It's totally doable. Tracking long-lasting disagreements and changing the way you look at them is a step towards repair and better connections. Walking through these processes, you gain a new perspective on just how connected everyone is and how those bonds can be strengthened. Push through the tough stuff and pave the way for a positive future—a place where **family** doesn't just mean people you're related to but people you can lean on.

Fostering Emotional Support Within the Family

Creating a **vibe** of emotional openness and support within your family means everyone can feel safe sharing their thoughts and feelings. It's all about building an **environment** where you can express emotions freely without fear of judgment. This requires a mix of patience, active listening, and empathy—like a warm, inviting space where everyone's feelings are valued.

Start by leading with **vulnerability**. Open up about your own feelings, even the hard or uncomfortable ones. Sharing moments of joy, sadness, frustration, or anxiety shows others that it's okay to be real. For instance, you might say, "I felt really anxious about work today," or "I'm so happy I got to relax with a good book." These small but meaningful shares set the stage for others to open up too.

It's also important to **validate** each other's feelings. When someone shares something, listen actively—nod, maintain eye contact, and offer words of support. Saying things like, "I get how that could make you feel bad" or "That sounds really tough" can make a world of difference. Even if you don't have a solution, showing empathy helps build that supportive atmosphere.

Now, let's talk about "emotional **coaching**." Think of it like having a guide who helps you understand and navigate your feelings better. Emotional coaching involves teaching family members how to recognize their emotions, articulate them, and respond healthily. It's like giving someone a helping hand on their emotional journey.

Start with yourself and model these behaviors. When you're feeling angry, don't just react; take a deep breath and say something like, "I'm angry right now because..." This isn't just about controlling emotions but understanding them. Encourage family members to do the same—ask questions that help dig deeper, such as "How did that make you feel?" or "What do you think caused that feeling?" It's like guiding them through their emotional landscape with gentle, supportive nudges.

Of course, it takes time and patience, so keep reinforcing these habits in small, daily **interactions**. Over time, your family can start seeing feelings not as problems, but as important signals that need attention and care. Think of it like coaching a team, where everyone's learning and growing together.

Switching gears, let's discuss the "Family Check-In" **ritual**. This is a simple yet powerful way to regularly touch base with everyone's emotional states. Think of it like a pit stop for your family's emotional well-being.

Gather together once a week, maybe over dinner or in a cozy setting, and take turns sharing how you're feeling. Ask questions like, "What was the highlight of your week?" or "Did anything stress you out recently?" It's important to make this a judgment-free zone, where everyone feels safe to speak their mind. Keep it light and encouraging, almost like having a mini-game night where everyone's a winner simply for participating.

Make it **consistent**. Whether it's a weekly thing or bi-weekly, letting everyone know there's a regular time to share makes it part of your family's rhythm. Over time, this ritual can become a pillar of emotional support, ensuring everyone feels heard and valued.

In short, building emotional openness, becoming an emotional coach, and committing to regular check-ins can transform your family dynamics. The aim is to create a home where everyone feels safe to be their true selves, knowing they're part of a loving, supportive team.

Practical Exercise: Family Communication Strategy

Understanding and fixing family communication problems is super important if you want to heal and create a positive future. Let's start with figuring out what's been going wrong in your family talks. Maybe there's a lot of interrupting or not enough listening. It could be that folks are quick to jump to conclusions or that people just don't feel heard at all. Jot down these issues as you see them. This isn't about blaming but about **figuring** out what's going awry.

Once you've pinpointed the main communication problems, choose one specific issue to tackle. Don't try to fix every problem at once. That's overwhelming and likely ineffective. Maybe the issue you pick is that certain topics always lead to yelling. Or maybe it's that someone interrupts before anyone else gets a chance to speak. **Focus** on just one of these concerns. It helps to write it down. This will keep you focused and clear-headed on what you want to work on.

Next, paint a picture in your mind of what you ideally want to happen with this communication issue. **Imagine** the perfect scenario where everything goes smoothly. How does the conversation flow? Are folks taking turns? Is everyone calm? Writing this down helps solidify your goals. It's about envisioning the best outcome so you have a clear target to aim for.

Now it's time to plan how you can address the problem. Create a script or key points to talk about the issue. This helps you stay on track. Think about what you want to say, how you want to say it, and what responses you hope to hear. Having a plan makes you more **confident** and keeps the conversation productive.

Before you dive in, practice this conversation with a friend or therapist. Role-playing can be invaluable. It lets you try out your script and see where it might go off course. Plus, feedback from someone you trust can be really helpful. They might point out things you hadn't thought of or suggest better ways to phrase your thoughts.

After you've practiced, choose a good time to talk with your family member(s). Don't spring it on them in the middle of dinner or during a busy moment. Set aside a quiet, unhurried time when everyone can **focus** on the conversation. Mention beforehand what you want to talk about, without going into the whole discussion right then and there.

Reflect on how the conversation went. Think about what worked and what didn't. Did you get your points across? Did your family member(s) really listen? Did you feel more **connected** afterward? This reflection is crucial. Use this chance to tweak your strategy. Maybe some points need to be clearer, or perhaps you need to adjust your approach next time.

Using these steps can **transform** how you interact with your family. Keep practicing, stay patient, and remember—it's all about steady progress, not instant perfection.

In Conclusion

This chapter offers **valuable insights** into transforming your family relationships for a healthier, more supportive dynamic. You'll find

practical tools to set boundaries, improve communication, resolve conflicts, and foster emotional support. These steps are crucial for creating a **harmonious family** environment.

You've seen the importance of setting personal **boundaries** within the family to protect your emotions and well-being. You've learned about "emotional enmeshment" and how it can negatively affect relationships. The chapter has provided practical **communication tips** to break bad habits and encourage better conversations among family members. You've also discovered ways to address and settle lingering family **disputes**, so everyone can move forward together. Additionally, you've seen how making emotional **support** a regular part of family life can increase trust and understanding.

By applying these strategies, you can make positive changes that enhance the quality of your family interactions. With dedication and patience, you have the potential to build stronger, more loving connections with those who matter most. Keep these tips in mind and create the **healthy, happy family** life you deserve. Remember, it's a journey, and every small step counts towards improving your family dynamics.

Chapter 9: Breaking Free from Limiting Beliefs

Ever wondered why some **beliefs** seem to cling to you like glue, no matter how hard you try to shake them off? In this chapter, we'll dive into the stuff that's holding you back. I'll share how these **limiting beliefs** have hounded me until I took steps to change them—and how you can too.

You might think, "Nah, I don't have any..." But trust me, you'd be surprised how many hidden **thoughts** shape your life. I'll help you spot those annoying, inherited beliefs you didn't even know were there. And I'll show you how to **challenge** that negative self-talk that's been dragging you down.

We'll even dig into family **stories** that keep you stuck and learn how to flip them on their heads. Imagine replacing your old, limiting beliefs with **empowering** ones—it's like turning a dusty attic into a vibrant living space.

Stick with me, because by the end, you'll have a practical **exercise** for reframing those stubborn beliefs. Ready to get started? Let's kick those limiting thoughts to the curb and unlock your full **potential**. It's time to break free and become the best version of yourself.

Identifying Inherited Limiting Beliefs

Ever feel like something's just **holding** you back, but you can't quite put your finger on it? Sometimes, it could be those **beliefs** you've picked up from your family over the years. These aren't just ideas you thought of one day – they can be passed down through generations and might be **stopping** you from reaching your goals.

So, how do you spot these sneaky beliefs that come from family trauma? Well, you need to start by paying attention to what you think is true about yourself and the world around you. Questions like, "Why do I think I'm not good enough?" or "Why do I fear failure so much?" can help you dig deeper. If a belief seems rooted in fear, shame, or doubt, chances are it's linked to some kind of past family experience.

Hang out with your **thoughts** for a bit. Reflect on the things your family has said and done throughout your life. Maybe it was a pattern of criticism or a constant reminder that success looks a certain way. Anything that triggers strong emotions could signal an inherited belief. Once you're conscious of these roots, you can start dealing with them.

Belief systems are basically the mental rules you live by. They act as a road map, guiding how you handle life's ups and downs. These beliefs aren't just dreams you came up with as a kid. They're shaped by how things went down in your family – the good, the bad, and the tough stories you've heard or witnessed. It's like starting life with a set of instructions that made sense in your parents' or grandparents' world.

Take a moment to picture this: your beliefs are like a **garden**. Some beliefs are beautiful flowers you care for, while others are weeds you didn't want but somehow grew. These beliefs dictate if you feel safe, worthy, and capable. So, if you're always thinking you'll mess up, it might be because those old family stories planted a 'weed' saying, "You're not enough." To change things up, you've got to figure out which beliefs are flowers and which are weeds.

Alright, let's move on to a tool that can really help – the Belief **Inventory**. This is a technique to list and look at your main beliefs, helping you see which ones are working for you and which are holding you back.

First up, grab a piece of paper or open a note on your phone. Start by writing down the thoughts that pop into your mind when you think about yourself, your abilities, and your goals. Don't overthink it – just jot them down as they come.

After writing your list, slow down and read each belief carefully. Ask yourself, "Where did this come from?" Was it something you picked up from your parents, heard from your uncle, or saw your grandma deal with? If it feels familiar, it likely didn't start with you.

Now, pick out the beliefs that are clearly not helping you. These are the ones making you feel stuck, scared, or unhappy. Next to each one, write down a possible new belief that could replace it – one that feels positive and empowering. For example, if you wrote, "I always fail," you might replace it with, "I learn from my mistakes and get better each time."

Change isn't going to happen overnight, and it doesn't need to. It's about slowly watering those new, positive beliefs and finding support along the way. Think of this inventory as the beginning of your journey to freedom from those old, hidden holds.

So there you have it – identifying inherited limiting beliefs, understanding where they come from, and starting a process of changing them using the Belief Inventory technique. It's like heading into unknown territories of your mind, figuring out what's been lurking there, and deciding to plant something good instead.

Challenging Negative Self-Talk

You know those **crappy thoughts** that sneak into your head, telling you you're not good enough? Well, spotting and squashing those thoughts is where **freedom** begins. It's like your brain has set up a bad radio station, and you've got to change the channel.

First, pay attention to your thoughts. Sounds simple, right? But really, catch those little bummers as they pop up. When you're feeling low, stop and ask yourself: what's going through your head right now? Write it down if you can, because seeing them on paper can make them less intense. It's like shining a light on a shadow.

Now, don't be fooled—those bad thoughts feel real. But just because you think them, doesn't mean they're true. Picture it like a **courtroom** in your mind. Thoughts are like lawyers making a case, but not every argument holds water.

Here's where understanding "**cognitive distortions**" gets handy. Think of these distortions like funhouse mirrors—they warp reality. Things like overgeneralizing, where one bad moment means everything is awful. Or catastrophizing, where you imagine the absolute worst case. Identifying these can help you see when the circus is in town upstairs.

Take all-or-nothing thinking. Maybe you ace most of your tasks but mess up one thing, and suddenly you're a total failure. Sound familiar? Catch these thoughts and remember they're just funhouse lies. Lesser-known distortions like "mind reading" will have you assuming what others think about you, and let's be real, your assumptions are often miles off.

Now linking to the "**Thought Challenging**" exercise. Once you've spotted the distortions, it's time to fight back. This exercise is like a friendly sparring match with those negative thoughts.

Here's how it goes:

• Identify the Thought: Catch the negative thought as it's happening. Jot it down.

• Challenge It: Ask questions like, "Is this truly the case?" or "What would you tell a friend in this situation?"

• Look for Evidence: Up for a detective role? Search for solid proof. Both for and against the thought. Often, you'll find much more against it.

• Find Alternatives: What other positive ways could you view the situation? Opt for a balanced approach instead.

Let's say you're thinking, "I'm horrendous at my job." After going through the steps, you might realize you've gotten positive feedback before, or you nailed past projects. Replacing that nasty thought with, "I've had challenges, but I've succeeded before," can make a world of difference.

A smooth sort of transition brings us to flipping the switch from those dark spots to finding new, positive thoughts. Kind of like benching the gloomy teammate for one who lifts you up.

Finally, let's dig into how you sustain this. Like working out or learning a new skill, **consistency** is key here too. Training your brain to think differently takes some repetition. You might feel awkward at first, but hey, practice makes better.

Positive affirmations also pack a punch. They're like motivational posters for your brain. You might start with something simple like, "I'm capable," or, "I deserve good things." Say it out loud, even if you feel silly. Words have power.

Changing self-talk is a **game-changer** in the fight against limiting beliefs. Think of it like nurturing a garden. Pulling out the weeds of negativity makes room for the flowers you really want to bloom. With awareness, a bit of patience, and practice, you'll find those old limiting beliefs losing their grip, and a brighter future opening up ahead.

Reframing Family Narratives

Let's chat about seeing family stories in a brighter light. Growing up, you hear tales about your family's past. These **narratives** shape how you view yourself and your relatives. But sometimes, these stories are full of doom and gloom, making you feel trapped. The good news? You can actually flip these stories around to see them differently. Instead of focusing on the hardships, look for **resilience** and strength in those same tales.

Take that story about your grandparents struggling to make ends meet. Instead of viewing it as just a tale of hardship, think about their determination. They worked tirelessly to provide for their family, showing grit and dedication. This simple change in **perspective** can turn that story into one of inspiration, rather than just struggle. It's pretty magical, honestly.

But sometimes, it's tough to do this on your own. This is where **narrative therapy** comes in. It's all about looking at these stories with fresh eyes. It's a tool that helps you see your family history in a less painful way. By doing this, you can separate your identity from these old, sticky narratives. It's super empowering.

Imagine you're carrying a heavy backpack filled with all your inherited worries and bad experiences. Narrative therapy invites you to unpack that bag and take a closer look at each item. You figure out what you want to hold onto and what you can let go of. It's like editing a book about your life, keeping the parts that have value while ditching what's weighing you down.

Now, let's dive into the nuts and bolts of the "Story **Rewriting**" technique. This is kind of like hitting the refresh button on those family tales. Start by writing down the original story as you learned it. Keep it as detailed as possible. Next, identify the parts of the story that are hurtful or make you feel bad. This can be tricky, but stick with it.

Once you have the original version and the tough parts singled out, rewrite the story. Shift the focus from misery to strength or from blame to understanding. Let's take an old family story where everyone seemed constantly at odds. Instead of focusing on the endless fights, revisit the story to acknowledge everyone's struggles and needs. Often, the **conflict** comes from places of deep unmet needs or fears. Highlight moments of care and togetherness that may have been overshadowed by the disputes.

Say your parents had constant money issues. Instead of highlighting the tension, maybe reframe it to show their teamwork in facing financial stress. It's not about ignoring the bad parts but rather highlighting the strengths and positives. By reconnecting with these narrative threads, you create a new, empowering version of the story that casts your family and yourself in a different light.

And just like that, with these tools in hand, you're not just healing—you're writing a more positive future for yourself. Old stories can't hold you back anymore. Not if you don't let them. **Rewrite** your history in a way that lifts you up and helps you move forward, free from the baggage.

Developing Empowering Beliefs

Believe it or not, growing new, positive **beliefs** is essential for healing and moving forward. There are plenty of ways to do this, but let's start simple. Have you ever thought about how your thoughts **influence** your life? It's like planting seeds; you tend to forget about them until they blossom. With some effort, these seeds can turn into beautiful, empowering beliefs that help you flourish.

So, how can you actively grow these new beliefs? Here are some ideas:

• Focus on positive affirmations. Look yourself in the mirror and tell yourself something good. It might seem silly, but it works. Words shape thoughts, and thoughts shape reality. So affirm something positive today.

• Surround yourself with positive people. If you're always around negativity, it's like trying to grow a garden in the desert. But supportive friends? They're like sunshine and water for your mind.

• Practice **gratitude** regularly. Find a moment each day to think about things you're grateful for. It's a quick mood booster and shifts your focus to what's good in your life.

• Read or listen to uplifting content. Whether it's self-help books, podcasts, or inspiring talk shows, consuming positive material helps replace old negative scripts with new positive ones.

Now, let's talk about belief re-patterning. Sounds a bit technical, but it's pretty straightforward. You've got patterns of thought that influence your actions and results, right? Belief re-patterning is about changing those old, limiting patterns to reflect positive, empowering ones.

How can you re-pattern those beliefs? There are several ways:

• Visualization exercises. Imagine yourself acting in line with a new belief. See it, feel it, live it in your mind. Eventually, it's easier to actualize.

• Challenge and replace negative thoughts. When a limiting thought pops up, don't accept it. Instead, question it and replace it with something more positive. Slowly but surely, you'll start thinking differently.

• Consistency and practice. No change happens overnight. You've gotta put in the work day in and day out to make those positive patterns stick.

So, how does belief re-patterning change your actions and results? It's like upgrading your mental software. Old beliefs are like outdated programs—they slow you down and hamper your effectiveness. But new, empowered beliefs? They're state-of-the-art and make you way more efficient and optimistic, leading to better decisions and successful outcomes.

Let's smoothly transition over to our next tool, Affirmation Creation.

Here's where it gets interesting. Affirmation Creation exercises aim to help you identify and strengthen positive beliefs. Sounds simple, but let's dig into the how-tos.

Here's how you can create powerful **affirmations**:

• Identify what you need to change. Place your focus on specific aspects you want to improve. Let's say you want more confidence. Clear enough.

• Frame affirmations in the present tense. Like "I am confident and capable." This tricks your brain to act as if it's already true.

• Add emotion. Don't just say "I'm successful." Say, "I am wonderfully successful and it feels amazing!"

Got your affirmation? Now, repeat it. Daily. In the morning or right before you sleep seems to work best for a lot of guys. Stick to it, align your actions with these beliefs, and watch the **transformation** unfold.

So we've covered growing positive beliefs, belief re-patterning, and finally, creating affirmations. These methods are simple but can create a huge **impact** on your life. With time, you can break free from those limiting beliefs and step into a more positive future. Feels freeing, doesn't it?

Practical Exercise: Belief Reframing Technique

Start by thinking about a **belief** that's been dragging you down. It might be feeling like you're not good enough or worrying that you'll always fail. Don't sweat it if it's not a huge belief; just pick one that's been nagging at you and messing things up.

Next, let's dig into the **proof**. Beliefs don't just appear out of thin air—they come from stuff you've experienced or seen. So, dive into that belief. What evidence supports it? Have people told you this, or have there been specific situations where you felt this way? Now, flip it around and look at evidence against it. Think of times when you've succeeded or people who've had your back. You might be surprised to find there's way more against the belief than for it.

Once you've got a handle on the proof, it's time to **think** differently. What are some other ways to see this belief? Can you reframe those failures as learning moments? Or maybe you're comparing yourself to others too much. Try to shift your viewpoint to something more understanding and hopeful. This step needs some imagination, but it's powerful because it breaks down the walls that the belief built up.

After rethinking it all, it's **replacement** time. What positive belief can take over the old one? Maybe it's that you're capable and learning every day, instead of just not being good enough. Jot it down. This new belief should feel uplifting and true, at least more true than the old one.

Alright, let's set up a game **plan**. This will help cement your new belief. What actions will support it? If you believe you're learning every day, maybe that includes reading a motivating book or setting small goals and crushing them. Create a step-by-step plan so you don't feel lost or overwhelmed. Small actions taken consistently can shift your mindset gradually.

Developing a reminder **system** is the next crucial thing. You need daily reminders about your new belief so it sticks. Maybe you set a daily alarm with a motivational quote. Or write affirmations and stick them to your mirror or computer. Whatever works for you, make sure you keep the belief front and center.

Lastly, **track** your progress. How are your thoughts and actions changing over time? Keep a journal where you note any positive changes or moments when the new belief feels real. Look back every week or so and see how far you've come. Seeing progress is encouraging and makes the whole process feel worth it.

By following these steps, you'll start to see **changes**. It won't be a magic switch that makes everything perfect overnight. But step by step, you'll get there.

So there you have it—a practical exercise to help you break free from the beliefs that hold you back. Give it a shot and see the difference it makes in your life. You've got this, man!

In Conclusion

This chapter has provided **crucial insights** into breaking free from limiting beliefs that may stem from family trauma. It explained how your subconscious beliefs are often inherited and how they can **influence your life**. By focusing on positive self-talk, reinterpreting family narratives, and developing new empowering beliefs, you can pave the way for personal **growth** and emotional **healing**. These steps guide you in recognizing and combating negative internal dialogues that hold you back.

In this chapter, you've learned about recognizing belief systems shaped by family trauma, what cognitive distortions are and how they perpetuate limiting beliefs, the importance of reframing negative family narratives in a positive light, methods for creating and reinforcing positive, empowering beliefs, and practical exercises to help shift from limiting to empowering beliefs.

You now hold the **tools** to turn limiting beliefs into empowering ones. Remember, the key to positive change lies within you. Apply these techniques to **transform** your internal dialogue and establish a more confident and empowered version of yourself. Let's aim to build a **future** free from the constraints of negative family beliefs, taking small, consistent steps towards a positive and fulfilling life.

Chapter 10: Building Emotional Resilience

Ever feel like you're constantly bracing yourself for the next wave? I get it—life can throw more blows than a boxing ring. But stick around, because this chapter is your potential **game-changer**. Imagine spotting a storm and, instead of panicking, feeling genuinely **equipped** to handle it. We'll walk through ways together to develop **coping** strategies, putting you in the driver's seat rather than the back seat. It's like tuning a guitar; small adjustments make a world of difference. You'll also see how strengthening **emotional** regulation can be your secret weapon, taming those wild swings that knock you off balance. Plus, nurturing **self-compassion** is essential—imagine being your best cheerleader instead of worst critic. And you know what? Creating a personal **support** system is clutch for building **confidence**. By the end, a practical **exercise** solidifies what you've soaked up. Ready to stir some curiosity and up-level your resilience? Let's do this.

Developing Coping Strategies

It's time to **tackle** stress and emotional triggers head-on. You know, life throws you curveballs, and sometimes just breathing isn't enough to keep the stress at bay. So, how can you deal with it all in a healthy way? Let's dive into a bunch of practical strategies that can help you **manage** stress better.

Exercise is a fantastic way to blow off steam. Whether it's a brisk walk around the block or an intense session of kickboxing, getting your body moving releases endorphins—those feel-good hormones—and can shift your mood. Or how about journaling? Putting your thoughts and feelings on paper can provide a great sense of relief. Write down everything that's bothering you. No filter. It's like talking to a friend who won't judge, complain, or interrupt.

Mindfulness and meditation can also do wonders. Simple practices like deep breathing or guided meditations can help ground you and keep your mind focused. Find a quiet spot, close your eyes, and concentrate on your breath... Sometimes, that's all you need to calm the storm inside. Creativity is another outlet, too. Pick up a paintbrush, knit, make music—whatever lets you express yourself. It's not about being perfect but about releasing what's inside you.

One more thing—don't underestimate the power of talking to someone. Whether it's a trusted friend, family member, or therapist, saying things out loud can make your problems seem smaller and more manageable. Sometimes, all you need is to be heard.

All these strategies help regulate those pesky emotions. **Emotional regulation** is about controlling your emotional responses—even when life gets tough.

But why is it important? Well, being able to manage your emotions boosts **resilience**. It means you can handle stress without falling apart. Imagine you're a ship in a storm. Emotional regulation is your ballast, keeping you steady no matter how rough the sea gets. Reacting without thinking might make things worse, so, learning to control those reactions is key.

There are a few tricks to this. For instance, pausing to take a deep breath when you're upset can give you a moment to cool down. Reflect on what's truly bothering you—sometimes the problem isn't what you think it is at first. Also, keeping a level head lets you respond better to challenges.

Now, let me introduce you to something super handy: the **Coping Toolkit** exercise. This exercise helps you gather your own stress-management techniques. Think of it like having a toolbox but for your mental well-being.

Start by listing all the things that make you feel good or bring you relief. This can include activities, people, hobbies—anything that lifts your spirits. Maybe it's listening to music, gardening, or spending time with your pets.

Then, write down a few methods to handle stress when it rears its ugly head. For example:

• Taking deep breaths

• Walking away from the situation for a bit

• Calling a friend for a chat

• Writing down your feelings

• Engaging in a hobby

Keep this list in a place you can find it easily. The minute you start feeling overwhelmed, you can pull it out and see what might help in that moment. Keep adding to it as you discover new strategies.

By combining these strategies, understanding emotional regulation, and having your Coping Toolkit ready, you prepare yourself to **tackle** stress in healthier ways. Stress and emotional triggers don't stand a chance when you've got such tools at your disposal!

You've got practical techniques now. Explore them, see what works best for you, and watch as you start handling life's ups and downs with more ease. In the next section, we'll dig deeper into another essential topic, but for now, give these strategies a go and see how they help you.

Strengthening Emotional Regulation

Dealing with **emotions** isn't easy. When they're strong, like a raging storm, they can shake you up. But there's a way to make handling them better. It starts with emotional **regulation**. Ever noticed how some folks seem calm even when things go south? It's not magic. It's a skill. To get better at reacting to strong emotions, you need to practice.

Think of it like building muscle at the gym. You show up regularly, lift weights, and slowly, you get stronger. Same goes for your emotions. The more you work on managing them, the stronger your emotional muscles get. Take a moment when you're calm to think about how you'd respond in stressful situations. When you plan your responses ahead of time, you're less likely to be bowled over when those moments come.

Let's link this idea of managing emotions to a bigger picture: emotional **intelligence**. This is understanding not just your own feelings, but those of others too. It's like having a radar that picks up on emotional weather, either calm seas or choppy waters. Imagine being able to predict and prep for emotional outbreaks. Pretty handy when dealing with family issues, with all their emotional baggage and history.

So, what is emotional intelligence? It means recognizing your own emotions, understanding what they're telling you, and realizing how they affect the people around you. High emotional intelligence involves being aware of emotions and handling **relationships** judiciously and empathetically. This can help immensely when you're healing from family **trauma**.

Here's an example: If someone in your family triggers you, instead of reacting instinctively, you pause. Take a deep breath. Acknowledge your emotion. Process it. Is it anger? Sadness?

Understanding your reaction helps in choosing a healthier response. You're not ignoring your feelings but dealing with them in a way that's easier on you and those around you. It's like being a steady ship, navigating through life's storms.

Speaking of steady ships, there's a technique called "Emotion Surfing." It's all about riding those emotional waves without spilling over. When a strong emotion hits, picture it like a wave arriving at the shore. It's powerful, but temporary. So you don't have to drown in it. Here's how you do it:

• Notice the Emotion: Recognize that a strong feeling is coming up.

• Feel it Fully: Don't push it away. Allow yourself to experience it, but keep your cool.

• Label the Emotion: Anger, sadness, frustration—give it a name.

• Observe Your Reaction: Notice what your automatic response is— maybe your heart races, or you feel a knot in your stomach.

• Stay with It: The key is to stay with the emotion without reacting impulsively. Imagine you're a surfer on a board, feeling the sway of the wave under you. You don't act recklessly or get swept away. You stay balanced. The wave will pass.

These steps let you ride through the emotion without being consumed by it. It's a sort of dance where you acknowledge the feeling but don't give it the steering wheel.

Tying this all together, building emotional regulation is like crafting a solid **foundation**. You practice handling your emotions better, understand emotional intelligence, and use tools like Emotion Surfing to navigate those intense moments. Bit by bit, you create a safe space inside yourself. And this space becomes your **anchor** in dealing with whatever family history throws at you.

That's it—the heart of strengthening emotional regulation. One small step at a time until you're mastering those **waves** instead of letting them overwhelm you.

Nurturing Self-Compassion

Let's chat about something truly life-changing: developing a kind and understanding **relationship** with yourself. Picture this: you're always ready to cheer up a buddy when he's down, right? But when it comes to you, that kindness often gets lost. Instead of a loving cheerleader, you get an inner critic, always ready with harsh words. It's time to change that.

Start small. Think of yourself as a friend. Next time you mess up, instead of berating yourself, say the kind words you'd offer someone else. This shift isn't magic — it takes **practice**. It's like building a muscle. Each kind thought, each gesture of self-affection, adds strength to that muscle.

Talk positively to yourself, especially during tough times. You can stow away those nagging thoughts and overcritical words. Replace them with **affirmations**. Things like, "I'm doing my best," or "It's okay to not be perfect." Simple yet impactful stuff. You can even get crafty and write these down or say them out loud — that's extra brownie points for self-love.

Moving on, let's explain what self-compassion actually is and how it helps with **emotional** healing. Self-compassion, in a nutshell, is treating yourself with the same kindness, concern, and support you'd show anyone you actually care about. Instead of constantly criticizing yourself for your failings, self-compassion involves acknowledging that making mistakes is part of being human. You make room for your imperfections without harsh judgment.

Self-compassion comes with three major bits — self-kindness over self-judgement, common humanity instead of isolation, and **mindfulness** instead of over-identification. Saying a comforting "It's okay and normal to feel bad sometimes" can work wonders for your emotional state. It makes difficult situations more bearable. Accepting your many quirks and errors without that extra baggage of shame speeds up the emotional healing process.

With self-compassion, you're not pushing away your pain but rather embracing it and understanding it's part of everyone's story. This acceptance builds emotional **resilience**. It's like going from having a thin, fragile shell to a flexible, buffered heart-space where bruises don't sting as much. You're no longer just surviving but actually thriving.

Now, let's put this into **practice** with a "Self-Compassion Break" exercise. Suppose you're having a rough day, ridden with errors and guilt. Instead of spiraling, this exercise can anchor you. Here's what you do:

• Acknowledge the pain: Recognize the distress you're feeling. Say to yourself, "This is a tough moment," or "This hurts."

• Remember you're not alone: Recall that suffering and mistakes are part of life. Silently tell yourself, "Everyone goes through this," or even, "I'm not alone in feeling this way."

• Be kind to yourself: Finally, extend warmth and care to yourself. Imagine giving yourself a comforting hug. Say something soothing like, "May I give myself the compassion I need," or "I'm here for you."

Even just a minute or two doing this can transform your outlook. It halts that spiral of negativity and gives kindness a chance to step in.

In conclusion, nurturing self-compassion is all about reversing that inner negative chat, replacing criticism with care, and realizing you're in good company facing life's messes. By showing up kindly for yourself, you're not just mending old wounds but creating space for a much gentler **journey** forward.

Creating a Personal Support System

Building and maintaining a **network** of supportive relationships is like creating your own safety net. You're not meant to do all this alone. You'll find that surrounding yourself with positive and caring people can make a world of difference when you're feeling down. Start with those who genuinely care about you—friends, family, neighbors. Think about this like assembling a puzzle; each piece counts.

It's essential to **nurture** these relationships too. It's not just about reaching out when you need something. Spend time with them, listen, and be there for them as much as they are for you. Relationships are a two-way street. Engage in activities you all enjoy, have regular check-ins, and be honest about your feelings. This builds trust and deeper connections.

And another thing, don't shy away from asking for **help**. Sometimes, you might feel the urge to bear it all yourself, but everyone needs a hand once in a while. Being open about needing support isn't a weakness; it's a strength. You'll notice those who care about you will be more than happy to lend a hand.

So, you've got your network in place. Now let's talk about a neat concept: social **buffering**. It plays a huge role in emotional resilience. This idea revolves around how having supportive people around you can protect against stress. Knowing someone's there for you can relax you—sort of like having an emotional cushion that softens life's blows.

Think of social buffering as your safety net. When life decides to throw lemons at you, these bonds help you catch the lemons rather than being hit by them. This sense of security can actually lower stress hormones and lift your mood. Knowing someone's got your back when times are tough can be a game-changer.

Now, how do you keep this social buffer strong? Keep in regular **contact** with your support system. Share your highs and lows, celebrate their successes, and be present in their trials. Quality, not quantity, matters here. A few good friends will do more than a ton of acquaintances.

Moving from this, let's talk about a handy method called the "Support **Mapping**" technique. This is your go-to tool for figuring out who's in your support network and how to strengthen it.

Start by grabbing a blank sheet of paper. Draw a circle in the middle and put your name in it. Around this, draw smaller circles with their distance proportional to how close they are to you emotionally. Include anyone who offers you support—friends, family, co-workers, even mentors.

Next, assess the connections. Think about how strong the ties are and identify gaps. Are there folks you haven't connected with lately? Would certain relationships benefit from more attention? Jot down some steps to strengthen these bonds. It could be as simple as a coffee date, a meaningful chat, or even just sending a text.

This mapping helps you visually see your support, so you know where to channel your **energy**. Not every connection will be super strong, and that's okay. The point is to recognize who's there and figure out how to maintain and improve these connections.

Putting it all together, building a strong support system requires time and **effort**. You gotta give a little, take a little, and appreciate the people in your life. And remember, mutual support enriches everyone involved. So, get out there—connection by connection, map out your network, and let that social buffer keep life's stresses at bay.

Practical Exercise: Resilience-Building Plan

Building emotional resilience isn't as tough as you might think. Why not kick things off by **gauging** your current strength level?

Start by figuring out where you stand. There are tons of self-evaluation tools online that measure emotional resilience. They typically ask about how you handle stress, deal with change, and bounce back from setbacks. Just answer honestly, and you'll get a sense of your resilience level. Easy as pie, right?

Once you've got a clear picture, it's time to **identify** areas that could use a bit of work.

Take a look at where the self-evaluation suggests you might be struggling. Maybe keeping your cool when things go sideways is a challenge. Or perhaps bouncing back from rough days isn't your forte? Make a note of these key spots. Knowing exactly where to focus helps in **charting** your path forward.

Now that you know where you're at and what needs fine-tuning, let's dive into the fun part—strategies.

Choosing ways to improve can be exciting. There are loads of options out there. Here are a few easy ones:

• Mindfulness practices. A few minutes of meditation daily can make a world of difference.

• Physical activity. Yoga, walking, running—it's all good for clearing your mind.

• Positive affirmations. Telling yourself uplifting things can boost your mood over time.

Pick three strategies that **resonate** with you. Don't overthink it, just go with your gut.

So, you've chosen your strategies. What's next?

Planning is key. If you don't **schedule** these practices, they might fall by the wayside. Maybe do mindfulness exercises every morning? Physical activity three times a week? Set a reminder on your phone for your positive affirmations. By having a routine, it becomes as natural as brushing your teeth—just something you do without a second thought.

But what if you get lazy or forgetful?

Hold yourself **accountable**. Tell a buddy or family member about your plan. Or maybe join a community group with similar goals. You can even use apps to track your progress. When someone else knows what you're up to, it's harder to slack off.

Now that you've kickstarted the plan, how do you know if it's working?

Keep tabs on your feelings. Jot down any emotional highs and lows in a simple journal or your phone's notes app. Over time, you'll notice patterns and be able to see improvements. It's awesome to look back and see how far you've come.

Plans often need a bit of tweaking to be perfect.

If a strategy isn't **cutting** it, don't be afraid to swap it out for a new one. Trying different things can help. In time, you'll find what truly works for you.

That's it. Break down the process, make small adjustments, and you're on your way to a stronger, more resilient you. No guilt, no stress—just gradual, steady **improvement**.

In Conclusion

In this chapter, you've learned **essential strategies** to build emotional resilience. To help you better manage **stress** and difficult emotions, this guide has presented valuable **coping tools** and exercises. As a quick recap, here are the key points discussed:

You've seen different ways to handle stress and emotional **triggers**. You've learned about the importance of managing your feelings to stay strong, and how having strong feelings isn't always bad if you know how to handle them. You've also discovered ways to be kind and **forgiving** to yourself during tough times, as well as steps to make sure you have supportive people around you.

Accepting and applying these lessons will not only help you cope with daily **challenges** more effectively but will also improve your emotional **strength** over time. Keep practicing what you've learned and always remember, you have the power to manage your feelings and **heal** from past hurts.

Chapter 11: Reclaiming Your Personal Power

Ever felt like you're living someone else's life? It's a strange feeling, right? I know—I've been there. This chapter is gonna **change** your world. You'll find it super **eye-opening** as you start reading through; it's not just pages, it's a wake-up call.

You might not realize it yet, but everything in here is about making you **strong** and sure of yourself. Imagine shaking off those tendencies to let others call the shots. How would that feel? All the stuff we'll tackle—well, let's say it'll help you stand tall, **confident**, and ready to make choices that matter to you.

We've got bite-sized **exercises** too; they're meant to make those "a-ha" moments stick. Trust me, this isn't just theory. This chapter's like a personal **trainer** for your mind—putting you back in **control**.

Ready to **reclaim** your power? Let's do this.

Assertiveness Training for Trauma Survivors

Let's dive into **assertiveness** for trauma survivors. One of the biggest steps you can take in reclaiming your personal **power** is learning how to clearly and respectfully say what you need. It's about finding that sweet spot between being passive and aggressive.

When you're assertive, you're direct but still respectful. It's not about pushing others around or letting them push you around. It's a bit like walking a tightrope, keeping your balance. You're standing up for what you need while still valuing the other person's needs too.

There are some techniques to help you with this. Setting **boundaries** is a key part. For instance, when someone asks you to do something, pause for a moment before saying yes or no. Think about whether it's something you want or can do. If not, it's perfectly okay to say so.

Practice also speaking up in small ways, like ordering at a restaurant. It sounds simple, but it's great practice. You get used to expressing what you want or what you don't, even if it's just choosing what to eat. Plus, you're helping yourself get comfortable with the act of making decisions and communicating them.

Now, keeping it smooth as we switch gears. How does all this tie in with the meaning of assertive **communication**?

Assertive communication means more than just speaking up—it's about how you say it. The goal is to express your thoughts and feelings directly but stay respectful. Retreating into silence as adaptation doesn't heal you. Starting with small things can help. Like saying, "I feel upset when my opinion is ignored; I need you to listen," instead of bottling it up.

Think of it as a bridge. You're connecting your inner world with the outer world. You're letting people know where you stand, but without setting the whole forest on fire. This style helps in healing from family **trauma** as it changes how you interact. When you've been through trauma, you might have learned to stay quiet to keep the peace. Breaking that habit, and learning to speak up, can be transformative.

Segueing naturally into the tools of an assertiveness toolkit. Let's focus on "I-Statements."

"I-Statement" is a handy formula for sharing your thoughts and feelings without blaming others. The classic formula looks like this: "I feel [emotion] when [situation] because [reason]. I need [what you need]."

Take for instance, "I feel hurt when you cancel plans at the last minute because I was looking forward to seeing you. I need you to let me know as early as possible if you can't make it." Notice it focuses on your feelings without accusing the other person. You're stating your needs clearly and why they matter.

Using "I-Statements" can really transform the way you **communicate**. It fosters more meaningful conversations, making it easier to sort out misunderstandings. It doesn't turn someone's simple mistake into a huge confrontation. Think of it like planting the seeds of better communication—over time, you'll see the growth in how people respond to you.

Wrapping this up, assertiveness is your best friend when working on **healing**. Saying what you need clearly, learning the essence of assertive communication, and employing "I-Statements" all help in standing tall. Taking **control** here helps you build a foundation of respect and empathy. Plus, it feels pretty great to own your voice. Keep practicing, you will get there!

Overcoming People-Pleasing Tendencies

Ever notice how you're always **bending** over backward to make others happy? It's something a lot of us do, often without realizing. People-pleasing may seem harmless at first. But when you constantly accommodate others, it's like giving away little pieces of yourself. You start feeling worn out and unappreciated. So, how can you spot and change this habit?

Start by looking at moments when you say "yes" even though you want to say "no". Maybe it's agreeing to work late, even when you're exhausted. Or constantly doing favors for friends who never reciprocate. Catch yourself in these moments. Ask, "Am I doing this because I want to, or because I fear what might happen if I say 'no'?" Sometimes, just smiling and nodding isn't worth the price.

Jumping from people-pleasing to understanding codependency can really help. Codependency is like a tangled web of unhealthy relationships and learned behaviors, often rooted in family trauma. It's when you tie your self-worth to others' approval. Think about growing up—for some, love was conditional, based on behavior and making others happy. That's where this codependency starts.

When you dive into your past, you might find **wounds** that need healing. Maybe you were always the peacemaker, smoothing over family conflicts. Or you swallowed your feelings to keep someone else happy. By spotting these patterns, you can start cutting those ties. Don't worry, though—recognizing and dealing with it takes heart and patience.

Talking about people-pleasing is one thing; figuring out your specific **habits** is another. Here's what I like to call the "People-Pleasing Inventory." It sounds official, but it's really just about paying attention to your actions.

• Do you often agree with others to avoid conflict?

• Do you feel responsible for others' feelings, even when it's out of your control?

• How do you feel after you do something just to please someone else—resentful, drained, peaceful?

• Can you say "no" without feeling pangs of guilt?

• Are your own needs often at the bottom of your list?

If you answered "yes" more than a couple of times, there's work to do. Practicing "No" is a good start. Try low-stakes scenarios first, like refusing another slice of cake when you're full. With time, tackling bigger things will become easier. Also, self-care isn't selfish. Martyrs don't make good role models. They're human, too, just like you.

Navigating through these concepts shows there's interconnectivity between people-pleasing, codependency, and family trauma. They twist through your daily habits unless you untwist them with attention and care. So, make these habits visible. Call them out. Shift your focus from accommodating to **reclaiming** parts of yourself. Interested in fences? Build them. Space on boundaries and balance, not on self-sacrifice.

Reclaiming personal power isn't an overnight fix—but it's worth every scar and every effort. Ready to spot and modify your habits? Start small, stay patient, and remember, you're enough just as you are.

Developing Self-Trust and Confidence

Let's chat about how you can start **building** your approval for yourself–because, honestly, nothing feels better than having your own back. Think about the times you relied on someone else's thumbs-up to feel good about yourself. All of those moments weighed down by asking, "Is this okay?" or, "Did I do this right?" Dump them. You'll swap 'em out for a good helping of self-assuredness and self-liking. This isn't a one-size-fits-all outfit. It's custom-fit for you, growing bit by bit each day.

Start with small **promises** to yourself and keep them. Like setting the alarm early in the morning and actually following through. Or sticking to that new hobby. With every small goal you tick off, you're painting a picture of reliability. Ha! You knew you could count on yourself.

Another nugget–turn off the negative self-talk. Replace "I can't" with "What if I can?" Be your own cheerleader, aware of any time you belittle yourself. Think like talking to a friend: full of support, offering encouragement, and laced with kindness for trying. The more you cheer on your successes and forgive little stumbles, the better you'll feel about taking chances.

Alright, feeling your value is seeded in believing in your own **capabilities**. Imagine this–every laugh-out-loud accomplishment and quiet win is a brick. Lay them wisely, and you'll get a solid personal powerhouse. Don't forget, believing in your abilities doesn't just sit pretty. It's about trusting your gut, going for what seems difficult, and proving you can. Every "Yes, I did it!" adds muscle to your self-trust. It's like a feedback loop. The more you do stuff, the more you believe. And the more you believe, the cooler stuff you tackle.

Think of it like riding a bike for the first time. Wobbly at first, right? But every pedal you take, makes you learn. Every second you're not flat on your back, you get **confidence**. That's precisely how believing in your skills works. Soon, even the craziest slopes are doable because you've got miles under your belt.

But hey, sometimes we all need a little extra push. That's where a handy visualization trick comes in. Find a comfortable spot, close your eyes, and see Future You standing tall and confident. Picture yourself facing situations that normally freak you out. Like delivering that presentation or starting a new exam. Future You handles it like a pro; calm, composed, rocking it entirely.

Bring forth your senses. Can you hear the applause, feel the pride, and see the smile? Imagine the Heart Racing Mix calming down as confidence soars. Open your eyes–for that moment, you actually drew from somewhere comfortable and powerful.

Switching gears, think of self-trust and confidence-building like a **garden**. Sprinkle seeds by fulfilling promises and affirming strengths. With steady care, you'll see sprouts of trust. Be ever gentle and believing in your everyday choices—that garden flourishes. Continue nurturing these qualities so you'll grow an inner sanctuary that can't be shaken.

So, here's to stepping into your **power**, bit by bit, both quirky and monumental. Self-trust doesn't grow overnight but oh, is it so worth **investing** in yourself consistently!

Making Empowered Life Choices

To really make **decisions** that match who you are and what you **believe** in, you've gotta be honest with yourself. Think about what's important to you and why. It's more about aligning actions with your core **values** and beliefs, rather than just going along with what others say or do. It's about knowing what makes you unique and sticking to it.

Start by asking yourself what truly matters to you. Is it honesty, kindness, freedom, or something else? When you know these things, it gets easier to make choices that feel right for you. Don't be afraid to say no to things that don't suit you. It's okay to put yourself first sometimes. Life's too short to be living according to someone else's script.

Idea of Personal Control

Gaining personal **control** is like finding the steering wheel of your life. When you're stuck in old family habits, it's easy to lose sight of your own path. Personal control helps you steer clear of these ingrained patterns. It's about making deliberate choices instead of just reacting to situations as they come.

It's about deciding how you want to respond to things, rather than just running on autopilot. It involves setting boundaries and sticking to them. This breaks your chains from past family habits. Think about a moment when someone pushed your buttons. Instead of reacting like you always do, take a step back. What if you chose a different reaction? Something more in line with who you are today?

To help make these conscious, strong choices, let's move to a little tool that can be super handy – the Decision-Making Chart.

Decision-Making Chart

Alright, here's how it goes. Imagine you're looking at a big decision and you need to feel confident about it. Grab a piece of paper and divide it into columns.

• **Options:** List out all the possible choices you've got. Don't hold back – even jot down the wild ones.

• Pros and Cons: For each option, list the good stuff and the not-so-good stuff.

• Values: Now, think back to those core values we talked about. How does each option stack up against what truly matters to you?

• Long-term Effects: Consider how each decision will play out in the long run. Is it something you'll be proud of? Will it cause regrets?

By doing this, you're giving yourself a clear picture of what each choice means for you and how it fits into your life. Sometimes just seeing it all laid out can make it easier to decide.

Knowing your values, asserting personal control, and using tools like the Decision-Making Chart all contribute to making empowered life **choices**. It's all interconnected – one bit supports the other.

Wrap up all Cases

Empowered life choices start with understanding and honoring your true self. Remaining conscious of your reactions and decisions frees you from the old patterns that might be holding you back. Tools like the Decision-Making Chart empower you to see choices from many angles and lead to decisions that align with your authentic self. Creating this connection of values, control, and clarity can steer you towards a **future** where you are in charge and can face life's twists and turns with **confidence**.

Practical Exercise: Personal Empowerment Statement

Let's talk about finding your **power** again. It all starts with understanding your main **values** and what you truly want. Think about it. What really matters to you? Is it honesty, freedom, family, being kind? List these things out so you get a clear picture. Imagine your life lined up with these values. This is key because knowing what you stand for gives you a direction, like a compass in a storm.

Once you've got your values sorted, figure out what you really **want**. Are you after inner peace? Success? Stronger relationships? When you nail this down, you're paving the road to your future. Jot down everything that crosses your mind.

Now, let's chat about taking back **control**. There are areas in your life that might feel wild, right? Consider your career, relationships, health, or even your own thoughts. Where do you feel stuck? Where do you want more control? Maybe it's your job that's making you miserable, or you feel sidelined in your family. Write these areas down. Narrowing these down will give you a clear focus on where to channel your efforts.

Alright, armed with your values and target areas, it's time to craft your personal **empowerment** statement. This is your promise to yourself. A declaration of how you're gonna live and grow. Think of it as a motivational note from you to you. Something like, "I commit to living my life with honesty and kindness, and I'll take back control of my career by seeking new opportunities." Make it strong and inspiring. This statement is like planting a flag on your desired ground.

But crafting a great statement is just the start. Next up, think about specific **actions** that back up your statement. What steps can you take daily or weekly to uphold this promise? For instance, if you mentioned seeking new career opportunities, maybe your actions include updating your resume, applying to jobs, or networking. Break it down into bite-sized tasks—things you can actually do. Make a list and get organized.

Sharing your statement with someone you trust can be really valuable. Find a friend or support person who gets it. Show them your statement and your list of actions. Why? Because speaking your **goals** out loud makes them real, and it also gives you someone who's on your side. This person can cheer you on or help you stay on track. There's power in community and accountability.

Now, don't forget to keep your empowerment statement visible. Stick it where you'll see it every day—on your mirror, desk, or even as a phone wallpaper. It's a daily reminder of where you're heading and what's important to you. Seeing it often will keep you motivated and focused.

Lastly, remember, you're always growing and changing. Life throws curveballs and you adapt. Regularly check in with your statement. See if it still resonates with you. Feel free to tweak or update it as needed. It's okay to evolve. Actually, it's great! Your personal empowerment statement should **grow** with you.

By following these steps, you're reclaiming your personal power, step by step. You're setting a clear path in a confusing world. You're not just dreaming; you're doing. So go ahead and take these steps seriously. It's your life—own it.

In Conclusion

In this chapter, you've learned about **strategies** and **techniques** to reclaim personal power through assertiveness, overcoming people-pleasing tendencies, and building **self-confidence**. These concepts and exercises are crucial for anyone seeking to overcome past **trauma** and make empowered choices in life.

You've seen valuable techniques for expressing needs and setting **boundaries** with clarity and respect. The importance of "assertive **communication**" in recovery from family trauma has been highlighted. You've also learned a straightforward approach for using "I-Statements" to express feelings and thoughts assertively.

Additionally, you've picked up tips for recognizing and adjusting excessive people-pleasing behaviors rooted in family trauma. Practical exercises for making decisions that reflect your true self and values have been provided to help you on your journey.

By applying these lessons, you can start making deeper **connections** with yourself and others, and steer your life towards a brighter, more empowered future. Keep practicing these **strategies**, and you'll see positive changes in how you interact with the world and take charge of your own happiness. Make every effort to own your personal power confidently, and shine brightly!

Chapter 12: Addressing Separation and Relationship Patterns

Ever wondered why some relationships feel like you're stuck in the same **loop**, over and over again? You might have thought it was just bad luck. But, you'd be surprised at how much your early experiences **shape** those patterns. This chapter is all about peeling back those layers.

You'll find yourself understanding how early **separations** can lay the foundation for your current connections. I'll help guide you through recognizing the core **language** you use in relationships—those things you say and think without even realizing it. Together, we'll explore how to **heal** attachment wounds, moving towards healthier relationship habits.

And here's where it gets actionable—you'll dive into **exercises** specifically crafted to analyze your own relationship patterns. Imagine shifting those ingrained habits to create **connections** that feel more genuine and fulfilling.

Ready to spark some real **change**? This chapter might just be what you need.

Understanding Early Separation Impacts

Imagine you were **separated** from your caregivers early in life. This kind of early separation can mess with how you form **relationships** as an adult. You might find it hard to trust or cling too tightly because deep down, you're scared they might leave. Maybe you feel a bit like you're on a rollercoaster, getting really close to someone and then freaking out, pushing them away. That's the shadow of early separation showing up in your grown-up life.

In relationships, it often means you're more on edge, worrying they might leave just like back then. You might **struggle** with being overly dependent or, on the flip side, keeping everyone at arm's length. This shaky start sticks with you, echoing in your romantic ties and even in friendships.

So why does this happen? **Attachment** theory gives us some clues. Developed by John Bowlby, it talks about how the bonds we form with our caregivers shape how we connect to others. There are different styles—secure, anxious, and avoidant, to name a few. If you had a stable, comforting attachment, you're more likely to be comfy in your relationships. But, that early chaos? It creates insecurities that hang around like unwanted guests.

Let's chat about attachment styles. If you're secure, great! You trust your partner and can count on them. But if you're anxious, you're always looking for reassurance. It's like you need constant proof that you're loved. And if you're avoidant, you act like you're too cool for deep connections, keeping things surface-level to protect yourself.

Why does attachment theory matter when trying to fix family **trauma**? Well, understanding your attachment style can help you see why you behave the way you do. It's a way to piece together the puzzle of your past and figure out how to construct healthier, happier relationships moving forward.

Okay, feeling curious? Let's jump into what I call the "Separation Impact" assessment. It's a little tool to help you figure out how those early experiences shaped your relationships now.

- Look at Your Relationships:

    - Do you often feel worried about being abandoned?
    - Are you quick to get jealous or possessive?

- Check How You Handle Conflicts:

    - Do you avoid arguments at all costs?
    - Or, do you escalate them quickly to feel in control?

- Reflect on Your Emotional Needs:

    - Are you always craving reassurance?
    - Is it tough for you to open up emotionally?

- Consider Your Independence Levels:

    - Do you find being alone scary or uncomfortable?
    - Or are you overly self-reliant, rarely asking for help?

By answering these questions, you're getting a clearer picture of how those early days still ripple through your life. Close your eyes for a second and think...What would it feel like if you weren't haunted by that underlying fear or worry in your relationships? Peaceful, right?

Understanding early separation impacts—plus using attachment theory to decode your past and this separation assessment to see how you've been shaped—gives you the tools to start **healing**. Isn't it nice to have a roadmap to a more secure and happy you? Don't stress. Everyone has their struggles. And recognizing the issue is the first step to fixing it. You're on your way to stronger, healthier **connections**—and navigating your relationships without the baggage.

Recognizing Relationship Core Language

You've probably **noticed** that your romantic relationships tend to follow some familiar grooves. Maybe you always seem to end up with the same types of problems or the same emotional hiccups. That's not a coincidence. Spotting these recurring themes and patterns can be quite an eye-opener. It's like having a **map** that shows where you've been and hints at where you tend to go.

Start by reflecting on your past relationships. Look for common threads. Did the same types of arguments keep cropping up? Were there recurring feelings of being ignored or misunderstood? Jot these down. This isn't about pointing fingers but about recognizing where things went sideways time and time again.

Think about the reactions and behaviors that you bring into relationships. Do you often feel like you're walking on eggshells or constantly seeking reassurance? These habits could pinpoint underlying fears or unmet needs that you're carrying from the past into your present.

Now, let's dive into a deeper idea: "**repetition** compulsion." It's a fancy name for a simple but tricky concept. This is when you find yourself repeating the same relationship patterns over and over without even realizing it. It's like your brain is on autopilot, steering you into familiar, but not necessarily healthy, territory.

Repetition compulsion is rooted in unresolved issues from your past, often stemming from childhood experiences or earlier traumas. Your mind tries to recreate situations that it didn't get right before, hoping to find a different outcome. The problem? You rarely break these patterns unless you're aware of them. And breaking free starts with recognizing that you're stuck in a loop.

So, what's next? Well, let's get hands-on with a "Relationship Pattern" **mapping** exercise. This exercise will help you see the recurring dynamics in your relationships clearly.

Grab a piece of paper and make three columns. In the first column, list the names of your past partners. Don't overthink it, just write them down. In the second column, note the most significant issues or conflicts you had with each person. Was it trust, money, emotional distance...whatever comes to mind.

In the third column, jot down your reactions and feelings during those conflicts. Did you feel abandoned, angry, belittled? Again, no need to get it perfect, just get it down.

Take a step back and look for **patterns**. Do you consistently attract partners who are emotionally unavailable? Or do you frequently feel underappreciated? These patterns are your relationship core language, the themes that are quietly shaping your romantic life.

Understanding these patterns is crucial. It's like having a cheat sheet for your emotional wiring. And recognizing these themes is the first step towards not letting them control you. From here, it's all about being **mindful** and, when possible, making conscious choices to steer your relationships in healthier directions.

In catching these patterns, in repetition, and doing the mapping, you're arming yourself with tools to make different choices. You're learning to spot when you might be on the verge of repeating a past mistake—an invaluable **skill**. Seeing things clearly is always the first move in making a change.

So, embrace the process. Write it down. And with each **discovery**, know that you've taken a step towards breaking those old, tiring patterns and crafting a new, healthier path for your relationships.

Healing Attachment Wounds

So, you've noticed that insecure attachment styles are kind of **tripping** you up. Maybe you find yourself **clinging** too tightly to people or pushing them away when they get too close. Either way, it's not fun, and it's affecting your relationships. The good news? There are ways to fix it.

One thing you can do is to **recognize** your patterns. It's like having a mirror held up to your face; you need to see what you're doing before you can make any changes. Are you acting needy? Or overly distant? Write it down, chat it out with a buddy, or discuss it with a therapist. Talking about it helps make it real, and from there, you can start to do things differently.

Next, **practice** new behaviors. If you tend to latch onto people, try giving them—and yourself—some space. Sounds simple, but it's tough. Like, when someone doesn't reply to your text right away, don't freak out. Instead, practice waiting patiently and doing something you enjoy while you wait. If you're usually the one who stays distant, challenge yourself to be a little more open. Share something personal or make a small gesture that shows you care. These little actions, over time, can change your overall patterns.

But remember, it doesn't happen overnight. Take small steps and be gentle with yourself. You're unlearning old habits and creating new ones.

Now, moving on from changing patterns, let's talk about "earned secure attachment." This is not about being born with a secure attachment style; it's about **building** it over time. The idea is that through consistent, healthy relationships and inner work, you can earn that sense of security you might have missed out on as a kid.

To get there, start by seeking relationships with people who are dependable and supportive. That could mean leaning on friends who always have your back or family members who offer unconditional support. When you experience consistent kindness and reliability from others, it chips away at those insecure patterns.

Another part of earning secure attachment is self-reflection. Keep a **journal** where you jot down your thoughts and feelings about your relationships. It might seem small, but this activity makes you more aware of how you're changing over time. Plus, it gives you concrete evidence that, yes, you are capable of forming healthy connections.

And here's a nice transition into creating a feeling of safety inside. This brings us to a helpful tool called "Secure Base" **visualization**. Imagine yourself in a place where you felt safe and loved. Maybe it's your grandma's house or a secret spot in a park. Picture every detail there: the smells, the sounds, the comfy chair, or the soft blanket.

In this visualization, see yourself being there with someone who makes you feel secure. Maybe it's a supportive friend or even an imaginary protector if that feels right. Spend a few minutes absorbing that feeling of security. Maybe you feel your shoulders drop a bit, or your breathing slows down. This isn't just daydreaming—it's training your brain to recognize and create safety.

Use this visualization whenever you start feeling anxious or uneasy in relationships. Over time, your brain will get better at returning to that secure base on its own. It's like giving yourself a little safety bubble you can carry around with you.

In summary, dealing with insecure attachments is about recognizing and changing patterns, building earned security through support and self-reflection, and practicing the secure base visualization. All these steps are pieces of a puzzle that, when put together, create a picture of healthier, happier **relationships**.

Creating Healthy Relationship Patterns

Healthy relationships are like well-tended gardens. They need the right balance of care, space, and structure to **flourish**. It's really about forming and keeping these healthy, balanced connections. So, how do you do it?

Take time to actually understand your needs. Not just yours, but those of the people you're connecting with. Knowing what you need from a relationship—whether it's lots of quality time, personal space, or open **communication**—helps in balancing different expectations.

Next, communicate. Seriously, my friend, talk it out. No one's a mind reader. If something feels off, it's okay to share that feeling. It creates **trust**. And trust is like the soil in that garden—it keeps everything grounded and growing.

Alright, let's connect this idea to an important foundation: **differentiation**. You've heard people talk about being their "own person" even when they're in a relationship, right? Well, that's what differentiation means. It's about being close to someone without losing your sense of self.

Why does it matter so much? Imagine you're on a dance floor. You don't want to step on someone's toes or be so far apart you can't dance together. Differentiation helps you keep your balance. It means you can be together without one overshadowing the other. You feel strong and independent, even as a couple.

Healthy differentiation involves a few key things: personal interests, space, and emotional independence. Make sure you're doing stuff you love, keeping some "you" time, and not relying entirely on your partner for emotional support. It creates a kind of dance where both parties feel free and connected, not trapped.

Now, let's ease into the nuts and bolts of making these ideas practical. A simple tool that's often overlooked is the "Relationship **Agreement**." It sounds a bit mood killer, but trust me, outlines like these can work wonders in setting clear expectations and **boundaries**.

Alright, here's a basic template to make a relationship agreement. You both sit down and fill it out together. It's kind of like building a roadmap.

Relationship Agreement Template:

• Your Needs:

• Daily check-ins to talk about your day

• A "no phones" rule at dinner

• Personal downtime each week to pursue hobbies

• Open discussions about finances monthly

• Support for each other's career goals

• Your Partner's Needs:

• Weekend time exclusively for family and friends

• Dividing household chores equally

• Limits on shared spending

• Flexible plans for vacations you want to take

• Regular date nights

• How You'll Handle **Conflict**:

• Take a 15-minute break if things get too heated

• Agree not to go to bed angry

• Listen actively and without interrupting

• Focus on resolving the issue, not winning the argument

• How You'll Support Each Other:

• Encouragements for personal goals by discussing progress

• Surprise acts of kindness, like little love notes or unexpected gifts

• Celebrating each other's achievements, no matter how small

Incorporate these ideas into your life and see how things start to shift. Healthy relationships aren't about eliminating problems but managing them better. Be open, differentiated, and clear.

And that's it, the way to those healthy relationship patterns. The journey is gradual—tiny steps like talking, understanding, and outlining your needs keep you and your loved ones in tune. You deserve these healthy, balanced relationships that enrich both your life and theirs.

Want to see **growth**? Keep tending to your relationship garden—water it with communication, give it space with differentiation, and structure it with agreements. It'll blossom beautifully.

Practical Exercise: Relationship Pattern Analysis

Alright, let's jump in.

First, think about your past **romantic** relationships. Yeah, I know, it's going to be a little uncomfortable, but trust me, it's worth it. Consider those important ones—the relationships that left a mark on you. Think about how they ended. Was it a break-up over a fight?

Maybe you just drifted apart? Could be someone moved away? It's crucial to keep these details in mind because you'll need them later.

Now that you've considered these relationships, let's move on.

Look at your mental list. Do you see any common themes or **patterns**? Maybe all your relationships ended because of similar reasons. Perhaps it was always about not having enough time for each other, or trust issues kept cropping up. Take note of these too. Common themes are your bread and butter here—they'll show you what might be going wrong repeatedly.

Alright, onto the next step.

Now, thinking about those patterns, consider how they might relate to your **family** history. Think about how your parents or family members interacted in their relationships. Did your parents argue about similar things? Maybe your dad was often absent, and now you find yourself fearing abandonment. Patterns can be really deep and trickle down from our early home life into our own adult relationships. Reflect on these thoughts; you're putting together the puzzle pieces of your relational life.

Here's a smooth lead-in to the next bit…

From the patterns you've spotted, pick one you really want to **change**. Maybe it's something like always attracting people who are emotionally unavailable. Whatever it is, this step's about prioritizing one major aspect you believe will bring a positive shift. It might feel tricky narrowing it down but focus on where you think you can begin to make real changes.

Taking the next step in stride…

With that one pattern in mind, it's time to come up with a **plan** to tackle it in future relationships. Think practically here. If it's about emotional availability, your plan might involve setting boundaries or asking more direct questions early on. Perhaps it's making a habit to identify red flags sooner rather than later. Your plan should feel actionable—after all, it's about creating a roadmap for healthier relationships.

And speaking of healthier relationships…

Trying out new **behaviors** to encourage healthier dynamics is a game-changer. This involves acting on your plan. Maybe you start practicing better communication or deciding to step back when a relationship shows early signs of familiar, unhealthy patterns. It's about being conscious and consistently applying those new tactics.

Last but definitely not least…

Regularly assessing the **approach** you've put into action is key. Regular checks on how this new pattern-breaking is working are important. Maybe every few weeks, reflect on any progress you've made or obstacles you've faced. Tweak what needs tweaking. Relationships are fluid, and as you learn more about yourself and others, your methods may need adjustments.

Stay patient and kind to yourself through this process. Changing relationship dynamics takes time, but each step gets you closer to the healthy, fulfilling **relationships** you deserve.

In Conclusion

This chapter offers **valuable insights** into how early experiences and relationship dynamics shape your current interactions. By understanding and addressing these factors, you can **improve your relationships** and emotional well-being. Here are the key takeaways to help you remember the most important points:

Your early **separations from caregivers** can have a lasting impact on how you form relationships later in life. It's crucial to understand the importance of **attachment theory** and how it relates to family trauma and healing. As you reflect on your romantic relationships, try to **identify recurring patterns** that might stem from these early experiences.

Learning strategies to **heal insecure attachments** can be a game-changer for your emotional health. By working on this, you'll be better equipped to create and maintain **healthy, balanced relationships** in all areas of your life.

Take these lessons to heart and put them into practice. By doing so, you'll gain a deeper understanding of yourself and the relationships around you. This knowledge, when applied, can lead to **stronger connections** and a more fulfilling emotional life.

Remember, it's not just about knowing this stuff – it's about using it in your day-to-day life. So go ahead, start applying these insights, and watch how they transform your relationships for the better.

Chapter 13: Creating a Positive Future

Ever **wondered** what's holding you back from the future you **crave**? I have, many times. Here's where this chapter steps in. It aims to **shake** things up a bit. You'll start to sketch out your healed self. Sounds cool, right? Then you'll get into setting **goals** that are more than just wishful thinking—they're in line with your true self. Like no more chasing someone else's dream. Will you confront your fear of success or happiness? Absolutely. It'll feel like pulling weeds in a garden—not easy, but so worth it.

This chapter also opens up new **possibilities** to shake things up in your life. No stone will be left unturned. And hey, there's a practical **exercise** too—visualizing your future self. You'll get a sneak peek of what's waiting on the **horizon**. Ready to make some real **changes**? Keep going, 'cause it's about to get good.

Envisioning Your Healed Self

Let's talk about creating a clear, exciting picture of your future, healed self. It all starts with being **honest** about what you really want in life. Think about the person you want to become, and imagine it in as much detail as possible. Does this future version of you have more friends? A new hobby? Maybe you're more at peace or feel more **confident**. You can jot these ideas down to make them more tangible.

Picture your mornings. What's your morning **routine** like? Do you wake up early, stretch, and take a moment to enjoy the quiet? Maybe you sip a cup of your favorite tea or coffee and plan your day with a clear mind. **Visualize** yourself going through your everyday tasks with joy and calm. See yourself dealing with challenges easily, without dragging past pains into the present. The goal is to create a vivid image that you can mentally visit and draw inspiration from.

Now, let's move from imagining to a more structured technique known as "future self-visualization." This is where you actively meditate or focus on seeing yourself as the person you want to become. Shut your eyes, breathe deeply, and see yourself in a setting where you're happy, healthy, and at peace. Try to make it as real as possible—what smells are around you, what sounds you hear, how your body feels in this ideal scenario.

Future self-visualization helps you grow because it gives you a clear **destination**. It's like knowing where you're going on a road trip. You can take different paths, but you know exactly where you want to end up. When you visualize your future self, you're training your brain to think that way. You start making choices that align with that **vision**. It's a way to believe in the person you aim to be, adding motivation and clarity to your daily actions.

Alright, let's put these ideas into words. This is where the "Future Self" journaling prompt comes in. Take some time, maybe a quiet evening or a lazy Sunday morning, and grab your journal. Answer this prompt: "Describe your perfect, healed future in detail."

Here's a guide to help:

• Where do you live?

• What does a typical day look like?

• Who are the important people in your life, and how do they support you?

• How do you handle challenges or bad experiences?

• How have you let go of past trauma?

• What achievements or goals have you reached?

Don't hold back—write it all down. Make this future as detailed and vivid as you can. It's like painting a picture where every detail tells a part of your story. You'll explore what you truly want and what **healing** means to you. Plus, it's like a sneak peek into how good things can be once you've dealt with your past traumas and emotional baggage.

By repeating this process, you'll reinforce these goals in your mind. Going back and reading your journal entries now and then can re-motivate you when you're feeling stuck or down. It's like having a roadmap to a better you, always ready and waiting.

So, give yourself permission to **dream** big. Think of all the wonderful ways your life can change when you're fully healed. Happy journaling!

Setting Goals Aligned with Your True Self

Let's talk about setting real **goals** that help you heal. Healing isn't a quick fix; it's a **journey** that asks for patience, understanding, and the right direction. Real goals should align with your true self—who you really are, not who others expect you to be. These goals help you feel seen, heard, and validated. They're about facing old wounds, shaking off the emotional baggage, and paving a better path for your future.

Think of this like planting seeds in a fertile field. You want to plant the right seeds—the ones that can really grow into something beautiful and strong. Real goals should feel like that: they should matter to you and make you feel alive. If you set goals that don't align with your inner truth, you'll end up feeling lost and unfulfilled.

To set these goals, start small. Ask yourself what you genuinely want. Test out a few goals and see how they sit with you—if they feel genuine. It's less about achieving perfection and more about moving in the right direction. It's about **progress**, not perfection.

Moving from there, let's dive into "values-based goal setting." Values-based goal setting is about anchoring your goals in the principles that matter most to you. Not what society values or what others think you should value. Picking goals based on your own **values** can be a game changer. It makes the journey feel worthwhile and fulfilling.

Let's say your values include kindness, honesty, and growth. Your goals should reflect these values. Maybe you set a goal to volunteer more because kindness is important to you. Or maybe you decide to pursue further education because you value growth. When goals match your values, each step toward that goal feels significant and rewarding. The fulfillment comes not just from achieving the goal but from embodying your values in the process.

To dig into this, grab a piece of paper. List out your top values. Next to each value, write down a few goals that align with them. You'll find that these goals not only feel right on paper but resonate deeply within you. They challenge you to live out your values every day.

Let's talk about checking if your goals are really supporting your true self. This brings us to the "Goal Alignment" checklist. A super handy tool to ensure you're on the right path. Here's a simple checklist you can keep with you:

• Does this goal align with my core values?

• Does it feel true to who I am?

• Will achieving this goal bring me a sense of fulfillment?

• Is this goal realistic and achievable in my current life stage?

• Do I feel passionate and excited about this goal?

If you can answer "yes" to these questions, then you're on the right track. If any of them give you pause, it might be worth reconsidering or tweaking that goal a bit. It's about small adjustments, not complete overhauls.

Having clear, aligned goals is **empowering**. It gives you a direction, a purpose. But more importantly, it respects who you are at your core. When you respect your true self, the healing process becomes genuine and lasting. These goals aren't just steps—they're meaningful strides towards a positive future.

With that foundation laid, you're better equipped to move forward with **courage** and clarity. Goals aligned with your values and true self naturally create a future brimming with possibilities. They help you shed the past's burden and stand tall, embracing a new, brighter path ahead.

Overcoming Fear of Success or Happiness

Sometimes, the hardest part about moving forward is the **fear** of what could happen if things actually go well. You'd think we'd all want good things, right? But deep down, there's often hidden resistance to these positive changes. Spotting this resistance can be the first step to breaking the pattern.

How can you tell if you're secretly resisting positive changes? Pay attention to little habits. If you're always finding reasons why you can't follow through with plans or congratulating yourself for only taking half measures, these could be signs. Maybe you get really close to achieving something awesome, and suddenly, something ridiculous happens to throw you off track.

Recognizing hidden resistance isn't a face-palm moment; it's just how some of us create an upper limit for ourselves. And, yep, this brings us to our next bit – the "upper limit problem".

See, the upper limit problem is that invisible **ceiling** you've built yourself. Gay Hendricks, the guy who coined the term, believes that you self-sabotage to not blast past this comfort zone. Maybe your family never achieved much success or happiness – so you've kinda become okay with that lifestyle. When good things start happening, it feels... off, even threatening.

Because of this invisible ceiling, your brain tries to push you back to "normal." So, let's talk about parents or grandparents who struggled and believed that **success** brought trouble. That belief can seep through generations, making you treat happiness or success as brief, scary moments destined to self-destruct.

Here's a smooth thought to ease you in – wouldn't it be nice to be okay with good things sticking around? This doesn't have to feel forced. You just need to get more familiar with success being, well, normal. Introducing: "**Success Desensitization.**"

Think of this like developing a taste for something new. Begin with modest doses. Small victories count. This means celebrating the little wins without downplaying them. You finished a project ahead of schedule? Treat yourself! This begins shifting your brain's notion that good stuff shouldn't last.

Create a list of achievable mini-goals and check them off as you go. This pleasurable pattern gets you comfortable with rewarding outcomes. Increase **challenges** gradually – like you'd eventually up your tolerance to spicy food by slowly raising the heat level.

Confide in someone or a group who absolutely dances when you win. Share the journey and cracked insecurities. They bring positive momentum, helping you retrain your thinking.

Focus on positive **reinforcement**. Let new patterns sink deep into your psyche. You start learning that fear of success or **happiness** is just smoke and mirrors, evaporating over time with gentle, consistent exposure.

Easing through the ideas from recognizing hidden resistance to understanding and tackling the upper limit problem, and finishing with practical techniques like success desensitization, you can allow yourself to grow more comfortable with all the good stuff coming your way. Your future self will thank you for starting this gentle, laid-back **process** now.

Exploring New Possibilities

Sometimes, it's tough to **imagine** your potential after years of dealing with family trauma. You can get stuck in a loop, replaying the same old problems. But trust me, there's a way out. Let's chat about some methods you can use to open up your mind and explore what's possible in your life.

Consider the idea of "post-traumatic **growth**." It's like a plant growing in harsh soil. You may have gone through some rough times, but that doesn't mean you can't grow stronger and better. Instead of just surviving, you have the option to **thrive**. Think about new skills you've picked up, or how you've learned to handle challenges. Maybe you've become more compassionate. Those strengths can actually set you up for a bright future.

So, how do you develop this post-traumatic growth? Start by recognizing your strengths. **Journal** about how you've changed in positive ways. Reflect on what you've learned and how those lessons can help you. Also, surround yourself with people who support you. Their encouragement can give you that extra push to move forward. Take small steps, like joining a new hobby group or volunteering. These activities expand your world and introduce you to fresh perspectives.

Now, moving on from recognizing growth... it's time to get creative. One way to start imagining a positive future is the "Possibility Expansion" **brainstorming** method. This isn't some rigid system, just a fun way to get those mental gears turning.

Grab a sheet of paper and a pen, or use your phone notes. Set a timer for ten minutes. During this time, jot down every possibility that pops into your mind, no matter how wild or unrealistic it seems. The goal is to spark **imagination**. Dream of everything from starting a new career to adopting a pet lizard. Seriously, anything goes. Once the timer dings, go through your list and pick out a few ideas that excite you.

Next, break those ideas into smaller, doable steps. If you're thinking about going back to school, maybe start by looking at courses online or chatting with someone who's a few steps ahead of you. Don't stress over making massive changes all at once. Tiny, manageable steps can lead to big transformations.

So, we've talked about opening your mind, developing growth, and you've started creating new ideas. But how do you keep the momentum? **Consistency** is key. Make a habit of revisiting your goals at least once a week. Check your progress, celebrate small wins, and adjust your plans if needed. Share your journey with a friend or counselor—they can offer advice and remind you of your progress when you can't see it yourself.

Each phase connects back to the others. Recognizing how you've grown builds a solid foundation. Brainstorming new possibilities lays out a roadmap. Stepping into action, no matter how small, drives everything forward. Keep the faith and stay consistent in nurturing these new paths.

In summary: the journey of healing and growing isn't always linear. But by acknowledging your strengths, expanding your possibilities, and staying consistent, you'll discover endless **opportunities** awaiting you.

Practical Exercise: Future Self Visualization

Let's talk about creating a fresh, positive future. It starts with opening your mind to new possibilities. This practical exercise is all about **visualization**.

Here's how to begin: Find a cozy spot and close your eyes. It's got to be comfy. Like your special corner or that one seat in the sunshine. Shutting your eyes helps you cut out the world. Lets your mind take front and center.

Next, picture yourself five years from now. But not just any 'you.' This is the you who has healed from family **trauma**. What do you see? Dive into the details. Maybe your smile is wider and your eyes sparkle brighter. Picture the people around you – friends, maybe even family who bring joy instead of pain.

Let's get even more specific with those details. Think about your **relationships**, achievements, and daily activities. Maybe you've built stronger connections, found new hobbies, or nailed that dream job. Notice the setting – is it a cozy apartment, a house filled with laughter, or calm surroundings surrounded by nature? Every tiny detail matters here because it shapes that future vision.

Pin down how you feel in that future state. Are you more peaceful, stronger emotionally, or physically fit? Get into your own skin, sensing every emotional shift. Do you feel lighter, maybe freer? Imagine mental clarity and a sturdier body. Emotions like confidence, joy, or even just contentment? Recognize those.

Start spotting key differences between your current self and this envisioned future self. What is it that makes Future You stand out? Compare **dreams**, habits, and attitudes. Maybe Future You is more outgoing. Or maybe you've learned to move on from grudges, making way for positivity.

Opening your eyes now, grab something to write with and jot down what stood out. Capture those important details of what you envisioned – the feelings, the scenery, the changes you've made. This note-taking helps anchor your vision in reality. Makes it sort of a tangible **plan** rather than just a fleeting thought.

To wrap things up, make a list of doable steps. Breaking it down into small, actionable **goals** is key. Maybe start with picking up a new hobby or reaching out to friends more often. Every task or habit change – anything that nudges you closer to that future version of yourself.

This visualization exercise is about guiding you step by step towards **healing** and transforming your life. Taking that time to imagine a bright, healthy, and happy future helps manifest it into your current life. Keep that vision close, and use it as **motivation** to take one step at a time toward the future you deserve.

In Conclusion

This chapter has given you a **roadmap** for envisioning and creating a positive future, breaking down complex ideas into actionable steps. By focusing on **healing** and setting clear **goals**, you can overcome obstacles like the fear of success and explore new possibilities in your life. Now, take the lessons you've learned and put them into practice to unlock a brighter, more fulfilling future.

In this chapter, you've seen the importance of having a strong **vision** of your healed self and the benefits it brings. You've learned how visualizing your future self helps in personal **growth** and goal-setting. You've also discovered why setting authentic and values-based goals is crucial for long-lasting fulfillment.

You've been introduced to techniques to identify and address **fears** that hinder your success and happiness, as well as ways to expand your sense of what's possible for your life after healing.

By applying these **principles** from this chapter, you can take charge of your healing process and steer your life towards a positive and empowered future. Keep these lessons in mind as you move forward, embracing **change** with confidence. Opportunities for a brighter future are within your reach—go out there and seize them!

To Conclude

The **point** of this book is to guide you from the constraints of family trauma towards a healing, liberated, and fulfilling future. You've come this far, committed to freeing yourself from inherited wounds and letting go of the emotional baggage of the past.

Let's recap what we've covered together:

We examined the nature and impact of family trauma on personal well-being, while also learning to recognize the signs and break the cycle of generational wounds. We delved into the epigenetics of trauma transmission, how neurobiological changes occur due to family trauma, and the roles of stress responses and the autonomic nervous system.

We focused on recognizing emotional inheritance, uncovering family secrets, mapping out your family's emotional legacy, and linking present struggles to past events. We decoded core emotional vocabularies, identified recurring life themes, inherited beliefs, and hidden family narratives.

You learned to pinpoint core complaints, descriptions, sentences, and traumas, culminating in a practical exercise to craft your core language map. We explored acknowledging inherited pain, letting go of generational guilt, and forgiving yourself and your ancestors, alongside practical exercises for emotional release.

We honed in on reconnecting with your younger self, addressing childhood wounds, using reparenting techniques for self-nurturing, and building resilience. You learned to set healthy boundaries, improve communication, address unresolved conflicts, and offer emotional support within your family.

We tackled identifying and challenging inherited limiting beliefs, reframing family narratives, and developing empowering beliefs. We discussed developing coping strategies, strengthening emotional regulation, nurturing self-compassion, and creating a personal support system.

You explored assertiveness training, overcoming people-pleasing tendencies, developing self-trust and confidence, and making empowered life choices. We covered understanding early separation impacts, recognizing relationship core language, healing attachment wounds, and creating healthy relationship patterns.

Finally, we visualized your healed self, set goals aligned with your true self, tackled the fear of success or happiness, and explored new possibilities.

What's next? Imagine a life unburdened by past traumas, where you embrace self-compassion, establish healthy patterns, and actualize your full potential. By applying the **techniques** and **exercises** from this book, you have the power to transform your existence, relationships, and overall well-being. Your **future** is not defined by past wounds but by the empowered choices you make today.

Start this transformative **journey** here:

Visit this link to find out more:

https://pxl.to/LoganMind

Join my Review Team!

Thank you for reading my **book**. Your thoughts and **insights** mean a lot to me, and I extend an **invitation** for you to join my Review Team. As a member, you'll receive a free copy of my book in exchange for your **honest** feedback. Your input will greatly contribute to the **improvement** of my future works.

Here's how you can join the ARC team:

• Click on "Join Review Team"

• Sign up to BookSprout

• Get notified every time I release a new **book**

Check out the team at this link:

https://pxl.to/loganmindteam

Help Me!

When you're done reading, I'd really appreciate it if you could take a moment to leave a review.

When you support an independent author, you're supporting a dream.

Your opinions matter greatly and have the power to influence future readers. **If you're satisfied**, please leave honest feedback by visiting the link below. Your **positive** words not only help others discover this book but also fuel my **passion** and dedication to storytelling.

If you have suggestions or ideas for improvement, kindly email me through the contact information provided at the link. Your **insights** are invaluable to me and I welcome your constructive criticism.

Alternatively, you can scan the QR code you'll find after selecting your book, which makes the process quick and **effortless**.

Your voice has a huge impact, and it only takes a few seconds. Thank you for your support and for being a part of this journey!

Visit this link to leave feedback:

https://pxl.to/9-hthfft-lm-review

Printed in Great Britain
by Amazon